Crohn's Disease and Colitis Recovery Guide

Artour Rakhimov

Dr. Artour Rakhimov

Disclaimer

TABLE OF CONTENTS

Introduction

This part 2 of the series "**Crohn's Disease and Ulcerative Colitis Books**" of 2 books. Part 1 of this series "**Crohn's Disease and Colitis: Hidden Triggers and Symptoms**" featured Chapters 1-4 which explained that currently there are simply no books and sources that provide even a list of specific signs of normal digestive health. The previous book analyzed these signs of the clean gut so that a person with IBD has clear understanding of goals and which symptoms to monitor.

These **signs of good digestion** include:
- no need for toilet paper due to the absence of soiling (i.e., no residue is left on the anus after a bowel movement)
- regular bowel movements
- absence of any offensive odor or smell from feces and absence of marks on the toilet bowl after a bowel movement
- ability to hold up to 1 liter (4.2 cups) of urine in the urinary bladder
- no need to perpetually consume pounds of yogurt, probiotics, and/or any other supplements or fermented foods due to the natural presence of good bacteria in the gut
- absence of biofilms on the lining of the gut that prevent absorption of nutrients and pollute the body with toxins
- absence of ear buzzing
- absence of unquenchable sensation of thirst due to recent GI exacerbation
- absence of moist nose
- warm feet and hands
- clean tongue (or absence of thick white or yellow coating on the tongue).

As the previous book explained these signs of healthy digestion and clean gut appear naturally when people improve their body O2 levels up to the medical norm (40 seconds for the DIY body-oxygen test)However, people with Crohn's disease or ulcerative colitis cannot increase their body-O2 content (it remains at about 20-30 seconds) due to digestive flare-ups or acute exacerbations. This happens due to hidden triggers that chronically keep the gut inflamed.

These hidden triggers include:
- food allergies to gluten, and possibly dairy, nuts, seeds, and other foods
- chemical triggers present in food and water (that include most spring and mineral waters, non-organic foods that contain fibers, essential oils, and many others)
- mechanical triggers due to abdominal pressure caused by bending, certain types of physical exercise (sometimes even walking after meals or on an empty stomach)
- allergic reactions via skin, air, and EMF fields ("dirty radiation")
- breath holds and certain breathing exercises that suddenly increase arterial CO_2 values.

Without knowledge of these hidden factors that are denied by modern medicine and gastroenterology, it is impossible to heal the gut. With this knowledge and avoidance of all triggers, it is possible to achieve no soiling (no need for toilet paper) an a few days and clinical remission for Crohn's disease or ulcerative colitis in 1-2 months.

The content of book 1 in this series is provided below.

1. Good and poor digestive health
1.1 Common symptoms of digestive problems
1.2 Signs of good digestive health (absence of digestive problems)
1.3 Causes of digestive problems and poor GI health
1.4 Body-oxygen test
1.5 Restoration of digestive health: the main goals
1.6 Expected effects of breathing retraining on common GI problems
2. Common triggers of digestive problems
2.1 Allergies
2.2 Chemical triggers present in food and water
2.3 Mechanical triggers
2.4 Allergic reactions via skin, air, and EMF fields
2.5 Negative effects of some breathing exercises

2.6 Synergetic effect of GI triggers
2.7 Sequences of negative symptoms for digestive flare-ups
2.8 Healthy villi and summary of putrefaction effects
2.9 Why does the gut react with diarrhea?
2.10 Effects of poor digestive health on body O2 and general health
3. Symptoms and signs to monitor
3.1 Commonly known symptoms
3.2 Frequent-urination log
3.3 Soiling effect
3.4 Ear buzzing
3.5 Unquenchable thirst due to recent GI exacerbation
3.6 Moist nose
3.7 Cold feet
3.8 Mental states
3.9 Body O2 monitoring
3.10 Why to record pulse?
4. Body weight
4.1 Effects of breathing exercises on overweight people
4.2 Effects of breathing exercises on underweight people

The present book (Chapter 5-16) provides the detailed plan for GI recovery.

5. Focal infections

It is only through considering the breathing retraining process that the full picture of the relationship between focal infections and chronic disease, including digestive problems, can be provided. Dr. Buteyko and his colleagues clinically observed, tested and developed their theory of focal infections.

The presence of focal infections interferes with the ability of breathing students to increase their CPs, normalize breathing, or even to recover from relapses of their digestive problems. The focal infections cannot be eliminated using the Buteyko breathing exercises and lifestyle changes. Moreover, due to the "rebound effect", the health of people who have focal infections may get even worse when the breathing exercises are practiced and higher CPs are temporarily achieved.

5.1 How dead tonsils prevent high CPs

The effect of dead or degenerated tonsils on one's digestive and overall health and CP is easy to understand using a practical example. Imagine a person with IBS or IBD, who starts with about a 10 second CP and raises it up to 20-25 s. His digestive problem is then under some control (with less soiling, more clear mind, better sleep and other effects) when his CP gets up to 20-23 s. But if this person has, for example, dead tonsils, further progress (beyond 25 s CP) would cause high-grade fever and throat pain with coughing, angina, and copious mucosal discharges. All these effects take place due to a severe reaction of the immune system, which tries to fight the bacteria and toxins generated in the dead tonsils.

The problem is that the degenerated tonsils have no normal blood supply and the immune cells in the blood cannot reach the pathogens hiding in his dead tonsils. As a result, the immune system creates inflammation in the surrounding tissues and the pathogens use this inflamed area to their advantage as a new breeding ground. That leads to infection and fever with heavier breathing and a sudden CP drop down to about 10-15 s. As a result, this student may again get more serious problems with IBS or IBD due to the fact that the focal infection in the dead tonsils became worse due to the higher CP achieved (25-30 s).

Dead tonsils can have an additional local effect due to toxins leaking from the tonsils into the throat and the digestive system. Many toxins, as with cavities in teeth in the next example, are very powerful in miniscule amounts. These poisonous substances have a direct effect on inflammation, ulcers, tumors, diverticula, strictures, and other abnormalities present in the gut.

This vicious circle (Breath work and better health → Higher CP → Tonsillar infection and fever → Low CP and recovery from the infection → Breath work and better health → Higher CP → Tonsillar infection and fever → Low CP …) can go on forever due to the rebound effect, even with application of other therapies (medication and antibiotics, throat gargling with best natural remedies, and many others). Some tonsils are not degenerated completely and can be restored with special techniques.

5.2 How cavities in teeth block the CP growth

As another example, imagine that a student has cavities in her teeth. This person can improve her breathing, and thus partially recover from a chronic health condition. When her CP rises up to about 30-40 s, her immune system can turn its attention to cavity-causing pathogens, but cannot defeat them since these pathogens reside on the surface of teeth with no blood access. More breath work leads to an even stronger immune response, but this enemy (cavities) is beyond the immune abilities. Therefore, no further progress is possible. The negative effects of tiny amounts of toxins leaking into the digestive system are sufficient to cause chronic GI problems. This focal infection does not have a strong rebound effect if the student maintains good or normal dental hygiene. (Poor hygiene with higher CP will favor the advance of cavities to other teeth and stronger inflammation in the gut.)

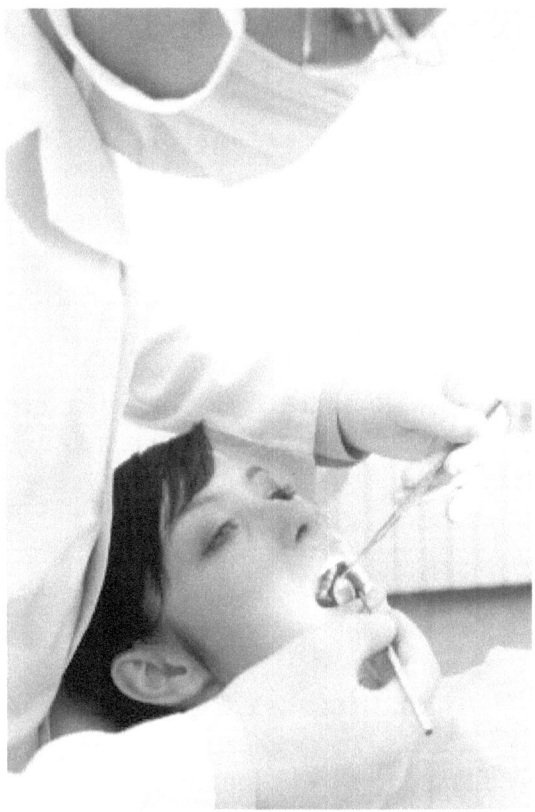

5.3 Effects of higher body O2 on foot mycosis (athlete's foot)

If a student has low CP (e.g., below 20 s), his athlete's foot infection usually remains dormant. While there could be an affected area between the smallest toes with light skin peeling, there is no redness, bleeding or feeling hot. This situation can be present for years. However, when his CP rises up to 25-40 s (even temporarily), mycosis of the feet advances to neighboring areas causing intense skin peeling, redness, deep lesions, bleeding and sensation of heat in the foot. The higher the CP achieved, the worse the spread of this fungal infection due to the same rebound effect.

This focal infection also produces a serious additional burden for the immune system that is constantly busy with fighting pathogens and tissue repair. Such an additional load makes digestive problems more resilient and can partially or completely prevent GI recovery.

5.4 Intestinal parasites prevent body O2 increase

The toxins produced by mature intestinal parasites (usually worms) intensify breathing regardless of the CP (immature parasites that do not lay eggs do not affect breathing to the same extent). Their negative effects depend mostly on their types and load, as well as their feeding cycles and food availability (when people fast, the parasites produce much less damage). Presence of intestinal parasites can restrict the CP to 20-35 s CP. Breathing exercises can increase the CP only for short periods of time.

Many types of worms feed in the duodenum, but reside in the lower parts of the GI tract. Their toxins worsen the flora in the gut and can also cause local inflammatory effects in the small intestine.

5.5 Effects of root canals on health and CP

This is the most unpredictable focal infection. It can be deadly for some patients or hardly noticeable depending on the personal health state and quality of periodontal work done. Properly done root canal treatment, with the right disinfection and correct sealing procedures, would probably not cause any big problems for a person who maintains moderate CPs (about 25-30 s) all the time. In this case, the immune system is strong enough to prevent the interaction of bacteria from dead teeth with other organs, while the toxins can be safely eliminated by the immune system from the organism.

However, since people with chronic health problems nearly always have less than 20 s CP, their root canals start to degenerate and interact with other pathogens present in the body. These processes can prevent their CP improvement and GI recovery. Their low CPs either don't improve or quickly drop down after breathing exercises.

6. Practical actions in relation to focal infections

6.1 Tonsils

If tonsils have been infected for several years, it is impossible to restore their functional abilities. In this case, tonsillectomy is necessary for breathing normalization, digestive improvements, and going beyond 25-30 s CP. Children and some adults who had infected tonsils for only 1-2 years can sometimes restore their tonsils using special conservative and prophylactic measures.

6.2 Cavities in the teeth

Regular visits to the dentist are important for general health. However, sometimes caries can develop in tiny cracks of treated teeth (between the filling and tooth) so that they are invisible even during dental examination, but still a very small amount of toxins are able to leak out. When a breathing student with about 20-35 s MCP tries to get higher CP numbers, he or she may notice that something prevents his or her further CP progress. The CP may rise slightly only for about 1 hour or less, or it may remain unchanged.

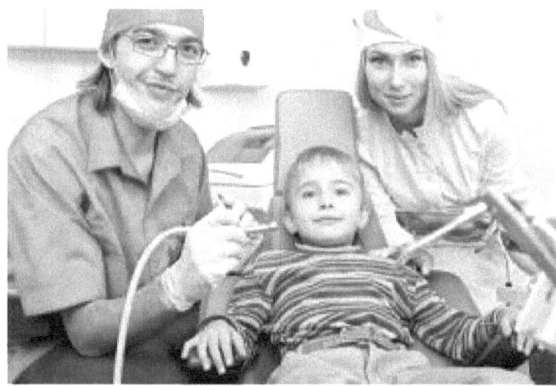

Here is a simple test to check for the presence of dental cavities. Gargle your mouth with a strong antiseptic solution (not with ordinary Listerine, but with more professional solutions used by dentists) for 10-15 minutes 3-4 times per day to suppress pathogens. Practice breathing exercises and monitor their effects. Follow this regime for 1 day. If your CP progress is stopped due to cavities, this "gargling" test will allow you to temporarily suppress the pathogens and achieve much higher CP numbers (e.g., 10 s more with the application of this method). If this method is applied for some days, some people can even temporarily break through 40 s MCP. If the use of this method does not yield any CP improvements, there are other causes for your CP deadlock.

6.3 Foot mycosis

Application of over-the-counter creams for affected skin areas and disinfection of all shoes and socks are necessary to deal with this fungus, which causes athlete's foot. There are now new creams available on the market. They have a double action and higher chance of success.

The cream is to be applied exactly as instructed: usually twice per day using a very thin layer, but for the whole affected area. The therapy should continue for some 5-7 days after all signs of the infections have disappeared. Natural remedies (including essential oils, garlic, hydrogen peroxide, grapefruit extract, alcohol, urine, and many others) have notoriously poor success rate against athlete's foot. Do not forget about your other shoes that can harbor spores of these fungi for months or years and infect you later.

6.4 Intestinal parasites

When the parasitic load is high, the student can easily notice that while she eats more food, she does not gain weight, but possibly even loses it. If this is the case, a family doctor can take fecal samples (2-3 more samples maybe required since many worms have cycles of laying eggs). Then either standard medication or some natural remedies can be used.

It is much more difficult to identify the presence of intestinal parasites, when there are only a few worms, which are not large in size. Paying attention to symptoms is useful in such cases. For example, activities of hookworms usually cause anal itching (since these worms lay their eggs at night near the anus), roundworms cause cold feet even at high CPs, etc.

6.5 Root canals

Some people, who have root canals, can achieve up to 2-3 min CPs without removal of their dead teeth. However, usually this relates to those people who do not have any serious health problems.

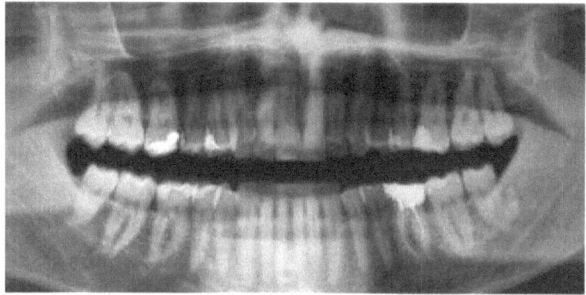

For people with long-lasting GI problems, the situation is usually different. When pathogens in the gut produce systemic effects (suppression of the immune system), these GI pathogens interact with pathogens due to root canals.

As a result, treatment of other health problems, such as gastritis, Crohn's disease, pancreatitis, and many other GI conditions, becomes impossible. The teeth bacteria, which are inaccessible, provide a support for other pathogens. The only way forward is to extract the dead teeth. Therefore, in cases of poor health, long-standing serious health problems or a weakened immune system, it is advisable to extract the dead teeth as soon as possible. Such students are usually stuck at lower CPs (about 12-15 s) and, while doing breathing exercises, these students cannot get even 2-3 s CP improvements.

A root canal generates toxins due to anaerobes and other pathogens living inside about 20 km of tiny tubules (former blood vessels of the live teeth). In addition, there is a dead-end of the artery leading to this tooth. When the CP is below 20 s, even temporarily, the tissues of this dead-end artery and the vein leaving the same tooth often become the source of infection and toxicity. Why?

During the root canal operation, the artery leading to the healthy live tooth is cut. As a result, the internal areas of these blood vessels become an excellent breeding ground for pathogens. The effect is much stronger at low CPs, while high CPs (over 30-35 s) will ensure quick tissue repair. These dead blood vessels themselves, at low CPs, become available to pathogens. Then the same pathogens can damage other blood vessels and cause appearance of the cardiovascular problems.

Several published studies found a link between root canals and increased incidence of the heart diseases (Mattila, 1993; Mattila et al, 2000; Dorn et al, 2002; Willershausen et al, 2009). In my view, the existence or appearance of any cardiovascular problems is a definite indication for immediate root canal removal. Only then is progress with breathing training and a higher CP more certain.

Warning. If in addition to your GI problems and a root canal (or 2 or more root canals), you have atrial fibrillation, myocardial infarction, or some other serious cardiovascular disease, you need to pull out your dead teeth as soon as possible.

6.6 Scraping the tongue

White or yellow coating on the tongue (that is present in people with IBD and nearly all ordinary people too) is not a classical focal infection. However, several studies proved that this coating is very toxic. Even some milligrams of these toxins are enough to cause digestive exacerbations.

Therefore, scraping the tongue with a plastic or metal spoon, or using a tongue scraper will help to reduce the toxic load and assist healing of the gut. This procedure should be done at least once per day, in the morning when most people have heaviest coating. You also need to check if you get it again later during the day. If you get it before lunch or supper, then it is important to scrape your tongue before other meals as well.

This factor alone can prevent GI recovery even if you eliminate all other triggers.

References

Dorn BR, Harris LJ, Wujick CT, Vertucci FJ, Progulske-Fox A, Invasion of vascular cells in vitro by Porphyromonas endodontalis, Int Endod J. 2002 Apr;35(4):366-71.

Mattila KJ. Dental infections as a risk factor for acute myocardial infarction, Eur Heart J. 1993 Dec;14 Suppl K:51-3.

Mattila KJ, Asikainen S, Wolf J, Jousimies-Somer H, Valtonen V, Nieminen M, Age, dental infections, and coronary heart disease, J Dent Res. 2000 Feb;79(2):756-60.

Willershausen B, Kasaj A, Willershausen I, Zahorka D, Briseño B, Blettner M, Genth-Zotz S, Münzel T, Association between chronic dental infection and acute myocardial infarction, J Endod. 2009 May;35(5):626-30.

7. Effects of chest breathing, posture, sleep and exercise

7.1 Chest breathing

Over 80% of modern people are habitual chest breathers. What are the effects?

The textbook, *Respiratory Physiology* (West, 2000), suggests that the lower 10% of the lungs transport more than 40 ml of oxygen per minute, while the upper 10% of the lungs transport less than 6 ml of oxygen per minute. As a result, the lower parts of the lungs are about 6-7 times more effective in oxygen transport than the top of the lungs due to richer blood supply. This effect takes place mostly due to gravity.

During thoracic breathing, the lower layers of the lungs, which are most valuable in oxygen transport, get much less, if any, fresh air (less oxygen supply). This causes reduced oxygen levels in the arterial blood and can lead to so-called "ventilation-perfusion" mismatch (as in COPD or emphysema).

Normal breathing is diaphragmatic, allowing homogeneous inflation of both lungs with fresh air, similar to what happens in the cylinder of a car engine due to the movement of the piston. During diaphragmatic breathing, all alveoli are homogeneously stretched vertically and get fresh air supply with higher O2 concentration for superior arterial blood oxygenation. In contrast, chest breathing creates problems with blood oxygenation.

Therefore, chest breathing leads to reduced cell oxygenation: the driving force for all chronic diseases, digestive problems included.

Dr. Shields, in his study, "*Lymph, lymph glands, and homeostasis*" (Shields, 1992) reported that diaphragmatic breathing stimulates the cleansing work of the lymph system by creating a negative pressure pulling the lymph through the lymphatic system. This increases the rate of elimination of toxins from visceral organs (digestive organs included) by about 15 times. Why is this so?

The lymph system, unlike the cardiovascular system with the heart, has no pump. The lymph nodes are located in those parts of the human body that get naturally compressed (squeezing) due to movements of body parts. For example, lymph nodes are located around the neck, above arm pits and groin area. Hence, when we move, stretch or turn the head, arms and legs, these lymph nodes get mechanical stimulation to push the lymph through valves. This is the reason for the movement of the lymphatic fluid.

However, the lymph nodes connected to the stomach, kidneys, liver, pancreas, spleen, large and small colons, and other vital organs are located just under the diaphragm - over 60% of all lymph nodes in total!

Hence, Nature expects us to use the diaphragm in order to remove waste products from the lymph nodes of all digestive organs all the time - literally with each breath, 24/7. Hence, another problem with thoracic or chest breathing is stagnation in the lymph system and accumulation of waste products in vital organs located under the diaphragm. As a result, chest breathing causes lymphatic stagnation in the digestive system and prevents its recovery.

From this view, it also becomes clear why breathing devices and physical exercise (especially with the Training Mask) are very beneficial for digestive health. These types of exercises are done with large ventilation rates (up to 100 L/min and more) and without CO_2 losses. In fact, CO_2 levels in the lungs increase during these activities.

Chest breathing usually naturally disappears when a person has more than 30 seconds for the morning body-oxygen test. Here are more details about the CP and chances of chest breathing.

Body-Oxygen Content	Automatic breathing at rest: diaphragmatic or chest?
1-10 s	Virtually always chest
11-20 s	Chest in over 90% of people
21-30 s	Mostly chest
31-40 s	Mostly belly
over 41 s	Virtually always belly

7.2 Poor posture makes GI recovery impossible

When the small intestine is inflamed, the passage of eaten food through the small intestine is already limited because of inflammation that includes swelling. Slouching further constricts certain areas (or folds) of the small intestine, prevents normal blood flow to GI organs and normal peristaltic waves. In addition, slouching leads to habitual chest breathing causing reduced blood oxygenation and lymphatic stagnation.

Slouching occurs due to low body-O2 content (usually less than 20 seconds). However, even people with about 25 s CP still have tendency to slouch.

When a person has over 30 s CP, slouching becomes less likely. And it disappears at higher CPs naturally, as is reflected in this Table.

Body-Oxygen Level	Minute Ventilation*	Chance of slouching
Less than 20 s	Over 12 L/min	Likely
20-30 s	9-12 L/min	Possible
30-40 s	6-9 L/min	Almost impossible
>40 s	<6 L/min	Virtually impossible

If you achieve over 30 seconds CP and try to slouch, your CP will drop down to about 25 seconds. I had breathing students who practiced a lot of physical exercise and, as a result, they could achieve about 30-32 seconds for the morning CP. However, still they were slouching during the day, their daily numbers were dropping down to only about 25 seconds. Once, they kept a straight spine during the day, their CP increased up to 30+ seconds.

Slouching decreases one's CP due to chest breathing, lymphatic stagnation and other effects. These effects are present in all people. In people with GI problems, the effects can be worse. Therefore, you need to learn how to have correct posture all the time, especially whilst eating and after meals.

One great option is to eat while standing. Computer work can also be done while standing. If you have a tendency to slouch while sitting, you can try to use a sitting ball or make a slightly inclined chair (with a small slope of about 5-7%), similar to an Alexander chair.

Magnesium deficiency is an additional factor that exacerbates this problem. People with low magnesium have a strong tendency to slouch, which disappears once they start using Mg supplements. Hence, make sure that you have enough magnesium in your diet. A lack of magnesium is the most common mineral deficiency present in modern people. Study how to conduct a 3-day test and later select the optimum amount of magnesium supplementation (if you need it) for higher CP and better health.

Summary. If you adopt those postures that are common in modern people, it will be impossible to defeat many digestive problems, such as IBD and IBS. You need to have a straight spine 2/7.

7.3 Sleep postures

For some people with serious GI problems, slouching during sleep can cause GI flare-up. The gut might be so sensitive that, in some cases, the best sleeping position is supine (on one's back), reclined or while sitting.

If you decide to sleep in a supine or reclined position, it would be smart to use one or two belts to prevent chest breathing during sleep. The main belt should be located on lower ribs (the lower part of the rib cage). It should be very tight so that it is difficult to insert a finger under the belt and it prevents any large chest inhalations. If you decide to use a second belt, it should be located 1-2 inches below the main belt to provide a slight restriction on abdominal breathing.

People with inflamed villi and chances of a GI flare-up should not position a belt on their navel (or the belly button). As we discussed before, additional pressure on the abdominal area can easily trigger a flare-up.

If you decide to sleep on the back or in a reclined position, in addition to 1 or 2 belts, you will also need to tape your mouth. Get the free manual "How to prevent mouth breathing" and follow its instructions for better sleep.

Sleeping sitting is a better choice since it helps to maintain higher morning CPs in comparison with any horizontal position. The main problem with sleeping sitting is discomfort. However, as a temporary measure (for some 2-3 nights), most people are able to tolerate or "survive" sleeping sitting.

If a person is unable to safely sleep on the chest or left side, he or she should try to partially repair his or her gut during daytime. Most people are able to recover their GI organs within 1 day to such a degree so as to sleep on the chest or left side without any problems.

7.4 General effects of sleep

Ideally, a person should have about 1-2 hours with no food in the stomach right before going to sleep. In order to achieve this, those people who go to sleep at about 11 pm can have a supper at about 5-6 pm and then a small snack later (at about 9 pm).

Note that going to sleep with too low blood sugar can have disastrous effects. You may spend up to 1-2 hours unsuccessfully trying to fall asleep. Having a small snack with carbohydrates, about 1 hour before going to sleep, quickly solves this problem. (A better long-term solution is to get over 50 s CP, or even higher numbers, that will help a person to be more flexible and tolerant to no meals or larger meals.)

For those people who exercise late (after work or at about 6-8 pm), late meals and hunger before sleep can be a serious problem. Then the solution is to find an exact (minimum) amount of eaten food that will allow you to fall asleep and sleep through the whole night without blood sugar drops. This amount of food should be digested before you go to sleep so that you have at least 15, better 30 minutes with an empty stomach before sleep. This will help you to slow down your breathing before falling asleep.

Those who have very low body weight can eat larger meals even 30-40 min before sleep without negative effects on their morning CP and quality of their sleep. In fact, they get even better sleep if they eat sooner before going to bed. They can go to sleep at the exact time when the stomach gets empty.

Somehow, if a person falls asleep in any horizontal position and there is still some food present in the stomach, hours of immobility during sleep have a large negative effect on biofilms and flora in the gut. (This effect is less strong for sleeping sitting.) As a result, eating late greatly worsens soiling and causes more frequent urination with reduced urinary volume. One solution to this challenge is to have a mechanical shaking of the body or the whole bed during sleep as when you have an overnight train, plane or bus. Then you can go to sleep with food in the stomach without any negative effects.

7.5 Sleep deprivation effects

When experimental animals are subjected to total and chronic sleep deprivation, they are likely to die, in about 2-3 weeks. The cause of death is a neurological stress combined with a lost desire to eat. Why do they lose a desire to eat? Even mild sleep deprivation worsens the production of digestive enzymes, the presence of healthy hunger, and flora in the gut. Therefore, getting sufficient sleep is very important for fast GI recovery.

There are many lifestyle factors, including fresh air and physical exercise during the day, that make quality of sleep much better.

One of your goals in relation to sleep is to create conditions when your morning CP is about the same as your evening CP. A small drop of 2-3 seconds is not a big deal, but if your CP drops by 5 or more seconds, you should review all possible causes that decrease your body O2 during sleep and find out which factors require corrections.

Keep in mind that with increased body-O2 content, people naturally require less sleep, make better food choices and have more effective digestion.

7.6 Exercise and running

Those people with GI problems, who do not tolerate abdominal pressure, need to avoid bending forward and twists to the sides. We discussed some of these problems above. What about running, swimming, playing basketball, and other activities and games?

Some people with inflamed villi are not restricted in relation to such activities and are able to run and jump without any negative effects. However, if someone has a duodenal or stomach ulcer (or some other structural defect), running or jumping can open the lesion and cause a GI flare-up.

What is safe for you is hard to predict. This depends on your current GI state. Also, the situation can change with time. For example, at one moment of time, running on a soft grass might be ok (if there are

animal products, such as meat, fish, dairy, and eggs. These extra nutrients and factors are:

- Vitamin B12 (cobalamin)

- Iron (in red meat and fish)

- A nearly ideal ratio of amino acids.

While many nutritionists and medical professionals are aware that vegetarian diet may suffer from low B21 and iron, and abnormal proportions in relation to amino acids, these people rarely notice that there is one amino acid, arginine, that is present in large amounts in animal products and is very limited in vegetables, greens, sprouts and lentils. Arginine is considered a non-essential amino acid for adults, but it is essential for children. However, when the CP is low (less than 20 s), the body may not produce arginine at all. Therefore, one will require dietary arginine. One of the main functions of arginine is to be used for production of NO (nitric oxide) that is probably a second most powerful vasodilator (after carbon dioxide). Vegetarian diets with low arginine content can affect body NO reserves.

It seems that this negative effect of low arginine intake is particularly strong in people who are genetically predisposed to heart disease. To my knowledge, there are no studies yet, but the idea makes some sense due to positive NO effects on the cardiovascular system.

The solution to this problem with vegetarian diets (reduced arginine intake) is to eat more nuts and seeds that are naturally high in arginine.

8.2 Fats

Requirements and correct amounts of fat (apart from fish oil) for each person depend on his or her body weight, CP, liver's and stomach's abilities to digest fats, lifestyle, current climate and daily physical exercise.

For most people, consumption and digestion of fats is not a problem. For people with GI disorders, it is more common to have problems with digestion of fats. This often happens due to liver problems and lack of liver enzymes. When some fat is not digested and makes its way pass the duidenum, this fat becomes food for pathogens. Blastocystis hominis is one of the common protozoal parasite that thrives on fats. Prolonged consumption of fats that are not digested by the body leads to overgrowth of this protozoal parasite. Common symptoms include diarrhea, nausea, abdominal cramps, bloating, greasy stool that is difficult to flash due to its floatability, excessive gas, poor mood, cold feet and anal itching.

Most cases of Blastocystis hominis infection become diagnosed as irritable bowel syndrome (even though one can easily notice large spherical species of Blastocystis hominis using an ordinary microscope). Larger CPs, together with dietary changes, exclusion of fats from the diet, and liver repair steps, allow fast elimination of Blastocystis hominis infection and greatly improved GI symptoms.

Which fats are better to eat? In the area of digestion, there are a few common rules, and I completely agree with a saying, "One man's food is another man's poison". Healthy people, with over 50 s CP, can generally eat whatever they find agreeable since they can trust their tastes. The situation with sick people is more complex, especially when digestive problems are present.

If the liver is weak, the fastest solution is to increase body O2, as Russian doctors proved in a clinical trial on people with liver cirrhosis and hepatitis B. Apart from the improved CP, it is beneficial for CP progress to create conditions for restoration of the liver and pancreas (see suggestions for underweight people above).

As about specific types of dietary fats, many people believe that cold-pressed olive oil and other cold-pressed unsaturated oils are best choices. However, due to their saturated nature, saturated fats are easier broken down by digestive enzymes and used by body cells. Common saturated fats include butter, coconut oil and palm oil.

Since Candida is a very common pathogen (even for those people who are not diagnosed with Candida yeast infection), one of the best fats against Candida is **coconut oil** which has caprylic acid, a powerful anti-fungal. Caprylic acid is sold as an anti-Candida remedy. Coconut milk and creamed coconut (brickets with a semisolid or solid white paste) are also good fat sources, especially for people with Candida yeast infection.

Butter is another great choice, for those who have no problems with digestions of fats. However, due to an abnormal state of the dairy industry, if you live in the USA, Canada, or Australia, consider using only organic butter since ordinary butter in these countries contain large amounts of pesticides, herbicides, hormones and antibiotics. Also, be aware about possible allergic reactions due to casein (main dairy protein) naturally present in butter.

Common margarines, even when they are based on unsaturated oils, have their own advantages. The margarines often contain an additive lecithin that helps to emulsify and digest fats. As a result, while margarines are considered by many doctors and nutritionists as a poor dietary choice, they are not that bad even for people with liver and GI problems. Margarines with hydrogenated oils should probably be avoided.

Keep in mind that, in the stomach, fats are digested last (due to their lower density in comparison with water and other foods). This means that no matter how thoroughly you chew your meals, fats are going to float on the top in the stomach, while others food particles will be digested along the walls of the stomach and moved down into the duodenum. As a result, the symptoms of fat malabsorption, if one has them, in the duodenum and further down the GI tract will be delayed.

8.3 Carbohydrates

Carbohydrates include simple and complex sugars.

Simple sugars, such as glucose, fructose and lactose, are found mainly in table sugar, cane sugar, nearly all fruits, honey, and some dairy products. The main problem with simple sugars is that people with many GI problems have Candida as one of the (main) pathogens in the small and large colons. As a result, nearly all fruits (avocado is ok) makes GI health worse. Raw honey and birch sugar Xylitol do not feed Candida. They can be used, but be aware of their light laxative effect. (Some people can get an inflammatory effect due to Xylitol.)

Millions of people enjoy fruits. However, if you have GI problems and your duodenum is not in a great shape (due to an ulcer, Crohn's disease, IBS, and so on), you need to stop feeding Candida or, at least, to find out if you have Candida overgrowth. It is very likely that fruits contribute to your poor health. How can you find out the effects of fruits and other simple sugars on your GI and overall health?

You can simply check, for 3 days, the effects of the diet that does not include simple sugars. Exclude fruits and foods with table sugar, glucose, or fructose from your diet. This will help you to temporary starve Candida. If Candida becomes less active, you should be able to notice improved GI signs (less soiling, and so forth). Nearly all my students who tried this **3-day no-fruit test** noticed greatly reduced soiling and other improvements in 1-2 days.

Complex carbohydrates are also able to feed pathogens. The key factor for better digestion in relation to complex carbohydrates is good chewing. The human body can digest up to 80% and more of starches in the mouth, but only if a person chews his or her complex carbohydrates very well.

8.4 Gluten

When the gut is already damaged or inflamed, gluten (a protein found in wheat, rye and other grains) acts like a sand-paper on the inflamed (i.e., damaged) villi located on the lining of the mucosal surfaces. Gluten wipes out or erases inflamed villi each time the person eats products with gluten (including bread, pasta, noodles, and so on). Even one piece of bread per day is enough to prevent gut restoration. Note that we are not talking about Celiac disease, but about a gradual conditioning of the immune system to a chemical that is too aggressive in relation to the inflamed or damaged lining of the GI tract.

These destructive effects of gluten on the inflamed duodenum are proven in clinical studies. In such conditions (a strong negative mechanical effect of gluten), the immune system virtually always gets conditioned to gluten. In other words, gluten also becomes a chemical trigger of the allergic reaction. A presence or appearance of this allergy can be confirmed using the allergy prick test. As a result, people with inflammation in the GI tract often (maybe in most or nearly all cases) develop an allergic reaction to gluten. This reaction can probably appear in some weeks after a person has inflammation somewhere in the GI tract. This relates not only to problems with duodenum, but also for those who have problems with gastritis or GERD.

As a result, in my view, every person with colitis, Crohn's disease, IBS, duodenal ulcers, duodenal cancer, gastritis, GERD, and other conditions that involve inflammation or structural abnormalities in the small intestine should avoid gluten during and after (for, at least, some months) GI recovery. Even in cases of diverticulitis in the large colon, blood in stool, and other GI conditions, elimination of gluten from the diet helps to heal the gut.

Note that, in most people with GI problems, presence of gluten in diet does not cause an immediate severe reaction. Gluten wipes out villi that later slowly putrefy in the colon. This leads to a greasy stool with an offensive smell, soiling, marks on the toilet, and many other negative effects. Therefore, they have a delayed long-term reaction.

As an alternative, you may try a 3-day gluten-free test and see the effects.

8.5 Fruits

As we discussed above in Carbohydrate Section, simple sugars from fruits feed Candida that is, nearly always, one of the pathogens that thrive in the damaged gut. As a result, many people are not able to repair their gut with daily consumption of fruits. Even 1-2 fruits per day are usually enough to keep biofilms and GI symptoms unchanged. (A lot of physical exercise with heavy perspiration helps to subdue Candida, but a temporary rest from fruit intake is useful and can be even necessary for faster GI recovery.)

Eating fruits can be resumed when a person has over 30 s CP 24/7 with no soiling and good perspiration due to exercise. However, even in these cases, one should be slow or gradual in increasing the amounts of eaten fruits. For example, one can eat 1-2 fruits for several days or even longer time, while monitoring soiling, urination, and other GI signs. Depending on the results achieved, one may increase fruit consumption later.

8.6 Dairy products

Negative effects of dairy are delayed and often mild. Therefore, these negative effects of dairy can remain unnoticed for many months. How to check if you are sensitive to dairy products or not? You can also exclude all dairy products for 3 days and see the effects. The problem is that, if there are any other remaining triggers, apart from dairy, then you will not find much difference. For example, if you eat gluten during this 3-day no-dairy test, gluten will spoil the results. If you have fruits every day, you will not be able to see the positive effects of your 3-day dairy-free diet. Therefore, you will need to exclude many other suspected foods and do other changes in order to be certain about the real effects of dairy on your GI health.

Some people can be fine with organic dairy, but not conventional one. Other people may find that they can safely eat organic milk yogurt, but cannot drink organic milk. The reasons for these numerous reactions are in the large number of potentially offensive substances that can cause GI problems. The possible triggers in dairy products are:

- milk sugar (lactose)

- casein (main protein in dairy products and milk)

- pesticides and herbicides (if dairy products are not organic)

- hormones and antibiotics (if dairy products are not organic and they are produced in the USA, Canada or Australia).

8.7 Soy products

Most soy products are not a right food for most, maybe all people. There are some additional substances present in soy products that cause a variety of problems.

- High levels of phytic acid in soy reduce assimilation of many minerals such as calcium, magnesium, copper, iron and zinc.

- Soy foods contain high levels of aluminum, which is toxic to the nervous system and the kidneys.

- Soy phytoestrogens disrupt endocrine function and may cause more problems with infertility and promote breast cancer in adult women.

- Soy phytoestrogens are potentially dangerous for the thyroid gland and can cause hypothyroidism and thyroid cancer.

- Trypsin inhibitors in soy interfere with digestion of proteins and may cause pancreatic disorders.

Studies show that the content of some harmful chemicals is reduced in fermented soy products. For people with GI problems, it is often useful to eliminate soy products for 3-5 days so as to see that the effects on their digestive health.

Soy yogurt may not cause any problems and even help in your GI recovery. If you buy it, you need to make sure that you get **organic unsweetened** soy yogurt. Some brands of soy yogurt even have inulin added to it. Inulin is a naturally occurring, indigestible and non-absorbable oligosaccharide that is produced by certain plants. Inulin has some prebiotic and potential anticancer activity. (Prebiotic properties mean that it is a food for probiotics. We will discuss this topic later.)

8.8 Sea salt vs. table salt

Sea salt is usually produced using solar evaporation from sea water or salt lakes. Production of table salt involves mining and use of vacuum pan evaporators for extraction of salt at very high temperature.

As a result, both types of salt have 98-99.9% sodium chloride with nearly the same sodium content. However, sea salt, due to more gentle production methods, has a higher mineral content, up to about 2%. For example, magnesium can be at the level of about 2,000 ppm (parts per million). Table salt has large amounts of iodine added (sufficient to produce health benefits) and aluminum (as anti-caking agent).

Even though nearly all people on the Earth consume salt every day, there are virtually no studies that compared health benefits and difference between these types of salts. After using medical search engines, I found only one such study research conducted at the University of Medicine and Dentistry of New Jersey, Maplewood. This study compared effects of tap water vs. distilled water and sea salt vs. table salt on blood pressure in rats over 4 month period of time. The abstract of this study is provided below.

Cystic Fibrosis

Flowers SW, Jamal IA, Bogden J, Thanki K, Ballester H, Hypertension induction in Dahl rats, J Natl Med Assoc. 1990 Dec;82(12):837-40.

University of Medicine and Dentistry of New Jersey, Maplewood.

There is experimental and epidemiologic evidence that some minerals and trace elements play a role in hypertension. We designed an experiment in which salt and water sources were manipulated to examine the possible impact of this relationship. A strain of rats (Dahl rats) known to become hypertensive with sodium chloride ingestion was used to study the effect of salt source and water source on the induction of hypertension. The group on tap water and table salt had blood pressures (184 mmHg +/- 19) significantly higher than every other group in the experiment. The experimental animals receiving tap water plus table salt had the highest blood pressure levels, although they consumed the lowest quantity of sodium. Analysis of the tap water samples showed "soft water" by analysis of calcium and magnesium concentration. This could adversely affect blood pressure. The relatively high magnesium concentration in sun evaporated sea salt may play a protective role in hypertension induction. The zinc and copper present in tap water may play an exacerbating role.

Soviet and Russian Buteyko breathing doctors suggested that sea salt health benefits are particularly noticeable in those people who produce large amounts of mucus (sputum or phlegm) due to presence of respiratory problems (such as asthma, bronchitis, cystic fibrosis, and so forth). Table salt, as these Russian doctors proposed, is not suitable for human consumption due to aluminum used as anti-caking agent and possible other causes.

These doctors did not discover any adverse effects of sea salt (even at large doses) on most people, including those with high blood pressure. Furthermore, since most of their patients reported better well-being when using sea salt, leading Soviet physiologist Dr K. P. Buteyko, MD, PhD, suggested to use additional amounts of sea salt (up to 1/2-1 teaspoon per day) every day for increased body oxygenation. They found that even people with severe gastritis, GERD and other digestive problems do not have any adverse reactions to extra sea salt if they follow certain rules. Here is the protocol.

Instructions: how to use sea salt

Dissolve 1/2-1 teaspoon of sea salt in a glass of spring or purified warm (or room temperature) water. Sip it slowly on an empty stomach when you start using it. Later, after 1-2 weeks, you can use it after meals or at any other time. You can also use more sea salt with meals. Additional suggestions are:

- People with serious kidney problems need to follow their specific guidelines related to daily sodium intake.

- People with asthma or inflammation of airways need to use warm water only.

- People with gastritis should sip water with dissolved sea salt slowly only on an empty stomach until they solve their digestive problems.

It seems that all evidence points out that table salt is not good for human (and rat) health as a food. It is much better to use only sea salt for our nutrition. Table salt can be used to make salt-water feet baths when one applies electrical grounding.

Many researchers believe that sea salt, when dissolved in purified or clean water, is able to restructure water forming clusters, while table salt does not have this ability. Some Buteyko practitioners heavily emphasize benefits of supplemental sea salt and nearly insist that their students should use additional sea salt every day.

There are possible added benefits of breathing exercises when one breathes through sea salt or rock salt while using the Frolov device or Amazing DIY breathing device to increase body-oxygen content, especially for people with problems including the lungs and airways or with excessive mucus production.

8.9 Water quality

When the gut is already a problem, water also becomes a factor that can either keep you sick or provide conditions for recovery. Nearly all US cities, as well as large cities in Canada, the UK, Ireland, Australia, and many other countries have poor quality of tap water. Tiny residues of several chemicals often have a significant negative effect that can prevent gut recovery. Some other countries (Scandinavia, Germany, the Netherlands, and so forth) have much better water quality.

In cases of GI problems, instead of tap water, you can use spring water. There are, however, many people with IBD who are sensitive to most types of spring water due to minuscule amounts of pesticides and herbicides (that contain aluminum). As a result, such people notice that nearly all spring waters make their GI problems worse. The best choice in such cases is to use **reverse osmosis water**, Evian and Volvic. These types of water have highest purity and quality. Note that there are many water brands that are produced with the use of reverse osmosis. This relates to Aquafina, some water brands for infants (often sold in separate sections in large US grocery stores and pharmacies), H2O (the brand name in Australia), and many others.

The safest choice for all people with ulcerative colitis and Crohn's disease is to use only these 3 types of water: **reverse osmosis water, Evian and Volvic**, while avoiding all other types of water including spring and mineral waters that claim to be super clean. In many cases, finding a local spring or source of pure water (coming from rocks) is also a suitable option. You may need to experiment with water and see what suits you best.

Keep in mind that negative effects of water can be delayed (up to 10-16 hours) and these negative effects (more soiling, more gas, bloating, etc.) can last for the next 1-2 days after you started to use suitable waters.

8.10 Honey

Honey is an excellent food for people with low weight, those who do a lot of physical exercise, and people with problems related to digestion of fats. Note that only raw honey does not feed Candida. Raw honey can also be labeled as "unpasteurized" or "extracted at cold temperatures". If there are no relevant labels, honey in health food shops is usually unpasteurized, while in conventional-food stores is heated. Whatever the case, it is still better to ask grocery people about their honey or to buy only those types of honey that clearly states that it is raw or unpasteurized.

Raw honey can be eaten as a first thing (before other foods) or separately. It has a mild laxative effect. Therefore, it can also be used by people with chronic constipation. Large amounts of honey (about 100 g daily or more) can cause some soiling, but no any other negative effects.

Some people can be sensitive to all types of honey and cannot recover their GI health without avoidance of honey.

8.11 Too high blood glucose

For people with existing GI problems, even 1-2 minutes of high blood sugar level produces a strong negative effect on their GI health. Somehow, increased blood glucose creates conditions favorable for pathogens that multiply, form biofilms, and generate toxins.

Among the very first signs of high blood sugar, in people with GI problems, are unquenchable thirst (on lips), feeling warm, and increased ear buzzing. Soon later, they notice increased urination with reduce urinary volume and lower CPs. Finally, for the next bowel movement (that can occur after or before the next meal), their stool becomes greasy (or more greasy) with more soiling. There are many other possible negative symptoms that we discussed above.

In people with GI problems, high blood sugar can have a double negative effect manifested in larger total urinary output. As we discussed before, a digestive flare-up causes inflammation and GI flare-up increasing water turnover and urinary volume. In addition, at over 10 ml/l for the blood glucose level, the kidneys tries to remove excessive glucose form the blood and increases urine production leading to even larger urinary output.

High blood glucose can appear due to a variety of reasons. The main cause is too low CP (less than 20 s), as in nearly all people with diabetes. The next factor that causes higher blood sugar levels is the circadian changes. As a result, many people experience high blood glucose in the morning: before the breakfast.

Another common cause of abnormally high blood glucose is a reaction to meals (so called "reactive hyperglycemia"). This effect usually occurs about 1-2 hours after a meal. Also due to circadian hormonal changes, reactive hyperglycemia is much stronger in the morning (after the breakfast), and becomes less prominent in the afternoon.

At higher CPs (about 20-30 s), people have much better blood glucose control both, in the morning, before breakfast, and after meals. However, 20-30 s CP is still not enough to prevent blood sugar increases and their negative effects on GI health. One needs to have about 35 s for the morning CP and even higher daily CP numbers (with good chewing) in order to avoid reactive hyperglycemia.

Even a slight daily increase in blood sugar levels (alone or as a single adverse factor) can make GI recovery impossible. Therefore, people with GI problems and excessive blood sugar fluctuations, should take good care about their blood glucose values. What are the possible solutions?

Smaller meals

In order to achieve normal blood sugar levels 24/7, one can have **smaller meals**. Assume that you found that an ordinary breakfast causes unquenchable thirst and other symptoms of high blood sugar. Due to an additional negative effect on inflammation in the intestines, a person is likely to have a reduced urinary volume for a single trip. Both these factors greatly increase urinary frequency.

If you found that, for example, your breakfast causes increased blood sugar levels, you can divide it on 2 or 3 parts. Note that with a strong hunger, the first half of your meal will be digested very fast (the stomach can be empty in 20-30 minutes).

Good chewing

Chewing food very well helps a lot with a better blood sugar control. With good chewing, a person is much more sensitive to his or her own satiety signs. Good chewing helps to notice these earliest signs when it is time to stop eating. How to chew foods, what the effects of poor and good chewing, and which foods require especially good chewing will be discussed in later parts of this book.

More fiber

Having more fiber and vegetables with your meals also assists in having better blood sugar control after meals due to slower digestion.

Foods with lower glycemic index

Some foods, due to a variety of reasons, release their energy slower and cause smaller blood sugar fluctuations. For example, corn meal, brown rice and buckwheat have very similar contents of starches and proteins. However, corn meal creates a largest blood sugar spike, while buckwheat the least. Beans and lentils cause smaller blood sugar fluctuations than the mentioned starchy foods. Finally, nuts have even smaller GI numbers.

You can find GI tables online and use them to plan your meals, if you suffer from or suspect that you have problems with too high blood glucose levels.

Important note. When a breathing student is slightly overweight (due to fat present on a belly) and he or she gets higher CPs, even small amounts of starches or fats can cause high blood glucose levels. This effect can take place in a large CP range: from about 15 up to 35, sometimes 50 s: In such cases, one solution is to avoid all starchy foods and fats (with possible exception of fish oil) or dramatically reduce the amounts of these foods, and have mainly vegetables in the diet. Better chewing will help here as well.

Chromium supplements (glucose tolerance factor)

For some people, taking chromium supplement helps to have a better blood sugar control.

Cooling down yourself and taking a cold shower

Imagine that you had your breakfast and in about 1.5-2 hours you start to feel warm and thirsty. You can reduce blood glucose by having less clothing, watering your arms and legs with cold water, or taking a cold shower for up to 2-3 minutes or even longer.

Spikes of high blood sugar can last for 10-30 minutes only. When blood sugar gets higher, in most people, the body produces more insulin that helps to drive excessive glucose from the blood stream into liver, muscle cells, and fat cells.

As mentioned above, even 1 minute of high blood sugar is enough to cause GI damage. Therefore, one needs to be pretty fast in these self-cooling actions.

8.12 Early years of life

Early years of life is an additional factor for choosing your optimum diet due to a better adaptation of the GI system to certain types of foods. It is true that most people can digest many types of vegetables, fruits, berries, greens, nuts, beans, lentils, and other food items that they never ate before. However, those foods that were eaten during formative years, up to teenage years, are often easier to digest. The body learned well and knows well what to do with familiar foods.

8.13 Major nutritional deficiencies

There are 4 major nutritional deficiencies in modern people:

- fish oil (or lack of DHA and EPA in the blood)

- calcium

- magnesium

- zinc.

These deficiencies appear and present due to 3 major factors:

- low body O2 that indicates poor perfusion of GI organs

- dramatic changes in a diet of humans during last 100 years

- high prevalence of digestive problems and other chronic diseases that impose additional requirements for many nutrients.

Many people are able to achieve normal digestive health without nutritional supplements. However, for most people, correct and minimum supplementation with these 4 nutrients helps to speed up their progress up to several times. There are also people who cannot progress at all without additional supplements, such as taking fish oil, Ca, Mg and/or Zn.

For more details, you need to know about how to conduct a 3-day test for nutritional deficiencies and define your personal requirements which also depend on your current CP level and GI state. This information can be found on NormalBreathing.com.

8.14 Major sources of pollution in modern people

Low body O2

When a personal CP is below 20 seconds, cells of the human body switch from aerobic to anaerobic respiration. This often leads to a generation of lactic acid (the normal value is about 1 mmol/L) and free radicals (incompletely oxidized products) with reversal of the Krebb cycle (also called the "citric acid cycle") and immunosuppression. This is the reason why getting over 20 s CP is a very important initial step to stop progression of many chronic diseases, including digestive disorders.

Abnormal GI flora

What are the main internal sources of pollution for modern humans? The human body harbors billions of viruses, bacteria, and other organisms living in different parts of the body. In fact, the total number of these microorganisms is greater than the number of cells in the body. Some of these microorganisms perform various useful jobs, but many others produce harmful or toxic substances.

Which region of the human body has the greatest number of these microorganisms? This is the large colon since about 50% of stool consists of bacteria and other microorganisms. If you have a normal GI flora (with no soiling), then the toxic load from the GI tract will be very small. However, since most people do not have normal GI health, their gut becomes a significant source of pollution.

Aluminum cookware

Avoid aluminum pans and other aluminum utensils. Use stainless steel and other safer utensils for cooking. Stainless steel is probably the best choice (if you do cooking) since it also provides some iron. (Iron-based utensils were the major source of iron for humans living centuries ago.)

Microwave cooking

The heating action of microwaves is based on resonation of chemical bonds between atoms. Microwaves generate mainly those electromagnetic frequencies, which resonate chemical bonds between hydrogen and oxygen (as in water), and hydrogen and carbon (as in fats). However, the intensity of electromagnetic impact for microwaves is high enough to break molecules into parts. This may not be a problem with water, but when some larger molecules are broken into 2 or more parts, they can become either useless or harmful (due to formation of free radicals).

Therefore, microwaves can be safely used for heating water or killing pathogens in toys, kitchen sponges and rags, but not for heating or cooking food.

Toxins coming with tap water and food

Tap water, as we discussed before, can contain many harmful chemicals. For people with digestive problems, these chemicals cause a stronger negative impact due to their direct contact with the surface of the GI tract.

Similarly, conventional (not organic) foods produce the same double negative effect (the systemic effect and the local one) due to the presence of pesticides, herbicides, nitrites, nitrates, hormones and antibiotics.

Therefore, you can accelerate your GI recovery up to 2-5 times, if you eat only organic food and use pure water. For some people (in cases of sensitivity to aluminum), transition to organic food and pure water can be a necessary factor for their digestive recovery.

Note that most types of spring or bottled water are not suitable for people with digestive problems. Safe varieties of water include "Evian", "Volvic" and reverse osmosis water.

8.15 Organic vs. non-organic foods

As it was discussed before, it is very difficult, in many cases impossible, to restore one's gut while eating conventional (or non-organic) foods.

However, those non-organic foods that have a very small amount of fiber are often well-tolerated by people with GI problems. This is because fiber is able to bind those toxic chemicals that are present in non-organic foods and that worsen inflammation and the state of the GI tract. These foods include:
- oils and fats
- fruit and vegetable juices
- wines and other alcoholic and non-alcoholic beverages.

Wild varieties of foods, such as seaweeds, wild berries, wild fruits, wild honey, and so forth are also free from harmful doses of toxic chemicals.

9. Chewing and soft diets

9.1 What are the key goals of chewing?

1. Chewing *mechanically breaks* solid and semi-solid foods into smaller particles.

The stomach and both colons do not have teeth. Therefore, they are unable to tear apart or separate even soft foods such as pieces of cooked vegetables or chunks of fruits. As a result, if one does not chew such foods well, their nutrients will putrefy in the large colon. This effect is considered in detail below.

2. Chewing *provides information* for the ENS (enteric nervous system) to better identify the incoming substances (to check if the body really needs them) and to prepare the appropriate enzymes for efficient processing down the conveyor.

When meals are well chewed, the chum slowly leaks from the mouth to the stomach. This process allows chemical analysis of the incoming foods. Existence of this process prevents overeating.

3. Chewing *chemically breaks* down food substances due to digestive enzymes produced in the mouth.

When food is well chewed, up to 80% of starches, 15% of fats, and 5% of proteins can be digested in the mouth, reducing the burden of digestion for the stomach, liver, and, especially, pancreas. More importantly, good chewing and digestion in the mouth prevent putrefaction of many substances, such as starches and proteins, in the colon.

4. With good chewing, it is *nearly impossible to overeat*.

It is easier to notice first signs of satiety. In some people, at certain moment of time, their saliva can stop flowing, and they cannot eat anymore.

9.2 Effects of poor chewing

When chewing is insufficient, some food particles remain too large and some chemical substances (especially starches) are not predigested. What are the effects of poor chewing?

- Many nutrients remain locked in their cells and become unavailable for the organism.

- Instead of providing nourishment, these large particles, with locked-in goodness, become a burden for the GI tract, causing more wear of the GI linings even for people who do not suffer from digestive problems.

- Worst of all, undigested substances and particles start to putrefy (rot) in the large colon, which has ideal conditions (temperature and humidity) for decomposition of nutrients, growth of pathogens, and generation of toxins.

Imagine what happens if you do not chew well enough. The proteins and starches from the eaten foods are doing to putrefy in the colon for many hours, until they are eliminated with a bowel movement. Of course, the body, especially at higher CPs, tries to get rid of this poisonous fecal matter. This can cause diarrhea or greasy stool with frequent bowel movements. We see that in such conditions (when soiling takes place), diarrhea is a protective reaction that reduces absorption of toxins from the gut. However, some of these toxins will still be able to penetrate into the blood stream night and day, causing various negative effects (brain fog, poor mood, cold feet, and so on). These toxins also constantly reduce one's CP, including the morning CP. Therefore, lack of chewing causes gradual and constant self-poisoning.

If the toxins from these small undigested amounts of foods are eaten all at once (imagine you eat only 1 gram of rotten fish or meat), then you can get signs of serious poisoning and end up in critical care. However, slow release of the same amount of your daily toxins (due to insufficient chewing) usually goes unnoticed. They poison the body 24/7.

I have had many cases when my breathing students managed to achieve no soiling in about 2-3 days just by better chewing. This is easier for those people who do not have serious digestive problems. However, if a person with Crohn's disease, duodenal ulcers or IBS is able to create the right conditions for gut recovery, he or she can also achieve no soiling in about 2-3 days with dramatic improvement in gut flora and reduced body pollution.

As a result, poor chewing is the main diet-related factor that leads to soiling (presence of fecal matter on the anus after defecation) and very poor digestive health in modern people.

9.3 Which solid foods do not require chewing?

If you swallow, without chewing, large chunks of raw, cooked or fried meat, fish, or eggs, these large chunks will be completely predigested in the stomach (with proteins successfully split on polypeptides). Let us consider this process in more detail.

When the walls of the stomach are in mechanical contact with food particles that are inside the stomach, the mucosal layers of the stomach produce hydrochloric acid and digestive enzymes that try to digest these food particles. This process can result in 2 outcomes: either the digestive enzymes reduce the size of these food particles (meaning that their digestion takes place) or not.

In the first situation, the ENS (enteric nervous system) is able to get information that food particles are yielding to chemical action of digestive enzymes. Then the ENS will make the stomach continue digestion until these food particles are completely predigested (or become a paste). This explains why the stomach will keep chunks of meat, fish, or eggs until they are reduced in size to a smooth paste.

However, if you swallow whole pieces of corn, whole nuts (cashew nuts or almonds), then the stomach will not be able to predigest them. (The predigestion of large pieces of nearly all types of food in the stomach is possible if you have over 90 s CP, but not when you have less than 70 s.) As a result, for nearly all people, whole pieces of corn or whole nuts will be pushed into the duodenum and they will make a long trip until they are eliminated with a bowel movement. (In fact, swallowing several corn pieces is sometimes used to define one's transition time, from the mouth until elimination with a bowel movement).

Whole pieces have a relatively small surface area. Therefore, these whole pieces can generate only small amounts of toxins when they putrefy in the large colon. The situation is much worse, if you chew a nut some 10-20 times and then swallow these tens or even hundreds of small pieces (each about 1-3 mm in size). These small pieces have a much larger total area and they can "successfully" rot in the colon and cause self-poisoning. The same is true when we swallow raw or cooked pieces of vegetables, beans, lentils, greens, and many other foods.

Therefore, people can safely swallow only large chunks of foods with a high protein content, such as meat, fish and eggs. Depending on their fat content, pieces of cheese possibly can also be digested in the stomach. But nearly all other solid foods cannot be digested by the GI system without good chewing. This relates even to many soft foods as well, such as grains of cooked rice, well cooked Broccoli, cauliflower or carrots, and ripe soft fruits (peaches, apples, mangos, papayas, and so forth).

9.4 Which liquefied foods do not require chewing?

Many foods can be transformed into a smooth paste, or a liquid or nearly liquid state. There are commercially available fruit smoothies, vegetable juices with pulp, vegetable pastes, nut milks, nut butters, and other products. In addition, one can use a blender to make a paste or smoothie from nearly any food. Do these soft foods require chewing?

If we review our previous ideas related to digestion of various nutrients, we can see that only starches can be and should be almost completely digested in the mouth, while fats and proteins remain almost unchanged after they are chewed in the mouth. Fats and proteins will be digested in the stomach and duodenum.

We can see that those foods that have large starch content should not be liquefied or, if liquefied, require good chewing. Therefore, smoothies and juices from most fruits and vegetables are relatively safe provided that one has hunger and digestive enzymes to take care of their good digestion.

However, foods that contain grains, rice, corn, buckwheat, potatoes, and other starches cannot be liquefied and swallowed with little or no chewing. Therefore, one cannot simply blend all his or her foods thinking that this will solve the problem with chewing and particle size.

What would happen if one blends an ordinary meal with proteins, complex carbohydrates, and fats and drinks it at once or even slower, in a few minutes?

As soon as this meal has starches, they are going to promote pathogens in the gut. This will worsen GI health and prevent GI recovery.

9.5 Which diet is best?

The answer to this question is simple. The best diet is one that naturally provides the human body with easiest breathing and maximum oxygen content without compromising energy level, ability to exercise and other parameters. However, if we consider practical life, the situation becomes very complex since people have very different digestive health and lifestyle. When a person has good digestive health (with no soiling after bowel movements, and other signs of good GI health) **raw vegetarian diets** provide many advantages. Such diet plans require minimum digestion while offering a wide variety of nutrients.

However, people with digestive problems are not able to tolerate many raw foods. As a result, their best diet is the one that helps to recover their GI organs. In many cases, when people have Crohn's disease, ulcerative colitis, IBS, other GI problems with inflammatory processes in the gut, they require **a gluten-free dairy-free soft diet** that is considered below. This diet can be called an "anti inflammatory diet" even though this phrase often refers to a diet that reduces inflammation in the whole body.

There are millions of naïve people who believe that the diet is the main factor that helps to reduce chronic inflammation.

In reality, inflammation is mainly controlled by 2 other factors: grounding (or electrical voltage) of the human body and tissue oxygenation. Inflammation becomes chronic if one's CP is less than 20 seconds. Inflammation starts to disappear when one has more than 30-35 seconds for the CP test. Earthing (grounding) is the key additional factor that helps to reduce inflammation and increase CP in those people who suffer from inflammatory conditions.

9.6 Why many people cannot eat raw foods?

If a raw vegetarian diet is the best choice, there should be reasons why ordinary people do not use these diets. First, most people have less than 25 seconds for the CP test. As a result, they naturally prefer (and enjoy) junk foods that include white flour and table sugar. Second, if an ordinary person tries to have a raw diet, he or she can create mechanical damage to his or her GI system. This happens due to one modern cultural habit that we discussed above: insufficient chewing. Raw foods, such as most vegetables, nuts, sprouts, and fruits, require very thorough chewing. But very few people chew foods well.

In conditions of fast eating or insufficient chewing, cooking makes vegetables and many other foods softer, increasing bioavailability of their nutrients and reducing the damaging effects due to mechanical friction and putrefaction of raw foods. In other words, when raw foods are not chewed well, their starches and proteins are going to putrefy in the colon, poisoning the body. At this point, we can consider good chewing in more detail.

9.7 Good chewing defined

Good chewing means chewing long enough so that you do not make any swallowing movements in your throat. In other words, the food must disappear itself due to slow leaking through a small gap (less than 1 mm in size) that exists between the tongue and mucosal surfaces of the mouth. If you chew food very well, your food becomes so small and watery (running) that it can move like a mucus from the mouth into the stomach.

Practically, if you try to chew soft ripe fruits (like peaches, mango, papaya, and apples) you may need about 40-60 chews per one small bite. If you take a teaspoon of brown rice or buckwheat, you may need up to 100-150 chews to make it disappear. If you have an average (or typical) portion of cooked rice, then it requires about 40-45 minutes of good chewing.

If you suspect or know that you do not chew food well, you can certainly check that good chewing greatly improves your digestive (and mental) well-being while increasing body oxygenation and improving overall health. Try it for 2-3 days and see the effects.

For people with digestive problems, chewing can become a single factor that predetermines their efforts to regain GI health. If you chew food very well, and follow other ideas described in this book, and get high CP (over 30 s) 24/7, your chances of digestive recovery are about 100%.

If you do not chew food very well, especially your starches, you will be unlikely to get even 30 s for the morning CP and your GI health will remain nearly the same. The only alternative to good chewing is to avoid starches (or follow those diets that avoid grains, corn, buckwheat, potatoes, yams, and other foods with high content of complex carbohydrates) and to cook or pre-blend vegetables.

A blender can be used to reduce chewing time of raw vegetables, sprouts and fruits. This method allows getting nearly all benefits of raw foods. Let us consider how you can benefit from a simple blender.

9.8 Using a blender to make raw meals

Spending 40-45 minutes chewing starchy foods makes meals very long. However, chewing time gets even longer if you also try to chew well raw vegetables, nuts, berries and sprouts. (When we eat cooked vegetables, there is no need to use a blender since cooking changes the structure of fibers, making them softer. Therefore, most cooked foods do not require a long time for chewing in order to be chewed well or until they become a paste.)

This problem can be solved by using the blades of a blender (or mixer), instead of our teeth, to chop or cut vegetables, greens, nuts, sprouts, berries, seeds, and so forth to much smaller pieces (but not to a liquid or paste state that requires no chewing since the GI system needs to know what is coming and how much).

You can pre-blend raw foods using the "Pulse" button of a blender. Here are the instructions.

First, you need to prepare a base. The base can be made from fruits only if you are ok with fruits. Blend 1-2 fruits (about 200-300 g or little more than 1/2 of a pound in total) for about 1 minute to make a smoothie. This is your base.

People with numerous GI problems, such as Crohn's disease, colitis, IBS, and many others have soiling and should avoid simple sugars and fruits, as we discussed above. If fruits are not for you at the present moment, you can use pure water. You will need the right amount of water. If you have too little water in the blender (and too dry mixture later), then the blades of the blender will not be able to grab and cut your pieces of raw foods. If you have too much water, the mixture will be too watery.

You can also use nut butters with water added or salad dressings as a base.

The next step is to put large pieces of vegetables, greens, nuts, sprouts, etc. in this liquid or semi-liquid base. Push the "Pulse" button for about 0.5 seconds up to 30-40 times, and you will get a semisolid mixture with particles up to about 0.5-1 mm in size. This meal does not require up to 100-120 chews to disappear in the mouth (remember that we should not swallow food at all). Then you can eat this meal in 10-15 min instead of 45-50 minutes. You will get a perfect raw goodness with all nutrients preserved.

The blender can reduce the time of chewing by about 3-5 or 7 times. This means that you will spend much less time for a meal that is based on raw vegetables, nuts, and sprouts: not, for example, 40-50 minutes, but only about 10-15 minutes of chewing.

With a little practice, you should be able to optimize the parameters and become fast in making such raw meals with a blender. Note that this raw meal should be eaten within 10-20 minutes after it is ready. You may store it in a refrigerator for later use, but the food will loose its great quality.

While these ideas (related to the blender) can be used by most people, people with inflammation in the small intestine cannot eat most types of raw vegetables and most nuts even if they chew these foods very well. Let us consider why.

9.9 Effects of raw foods on the inflamed gut

If you observe a drop of water on a skin of an apple or tomato, you will notice that the drop stays compact and does not spread over the surface of these types of produce. However, the inner parts of apples and tomatoes easily attract a lot of water. What are the causes of these large differences?

Fibers have different properties or abilities in relation to attraction of water molecules. Molecules of some fibers are more polarized and, as a result, these types of fibers attract many layers of water since water molecules are also polarized. Some other types of fibers have less polarized molecules. When water molecules are located on such un-polarized fibers, water molecules prefer to stay together rather than to spread over the surface of the "not-attractive" fiber. This is exactly what we observe on skins of apples or tomatoes.

Researchers say that there are about 4-7 different types of fibers. Leaves of most trees and bushes and skins of many vegetables and fruits repel water molecules. Such fibers are usually crispy if you try to chew them.

Some other fibers can attract a lot of water. For example, psyllium husks easily draw a very large amount of water. These types of fibers can be covered by several layers of water molecules due to their polarized chemical structure.

This ability to attract water often correlates with softness of the fibers.

When these fibers are in the damaged small colon, they produce different effects on the inflamed villi. Crispy types of fibers can easily damage (mechanically) or cut inflamed villi that are already weakened due to inflammation. What is the reason? These harsh fibers do not have a cushion (layers of water) on their surface. Therefore, these fibers can be destructive for the inflamed villi.

The soluble types of fibers are different since they are covered by layers of water molecules. These layers of water act as a cushion to reduce the mechanical impact and prevent additional mechanical damage caused by peristalsis. As a result of their gentle stimulation, the inflamed villi have chances to mature and recover.

Therefore, if a person with an inflamed small intestine eats raw foods (or skin of vegetables and greens) every day, he or she constantly creates additional damage that destroy villi and does not allow them to mature and become resilient to ordinary foods.

The solution to this problem is to eat only those foods that do not cause additional mechanical damage. Vegetables need to be cooked and chewed very well. Note that cooking changes the structure of some fibers only to some degree. It does not matter how long you cook green peppers, cabbage, or leaves of kale. They will still remain too harsh for the inflamed villi. The same is true for many other vegetables.

10 The anti-inflammatory diet

In this book, the notion "the anti-inflammatory diet" implies something that is very soft or of nearly paste-like consistency (as soft as sour cream or baby food) and also not irritating for the inflamed villi. For some people, it may sound like a "soft diet" or a "liquid diet". However, if you look at examples or lists of foods commonly suggested for the soft diet and liquid diet, you can easily discover that these diets are unsuitable for many people with chronic digestive problems due to the presence of simple sugars from fruits or gluten.

The anti-inflammatory diet is a temporary and necessary solution for the damaged or inflamed gut. Raw foods have a negative impact due to two different mechanisms. First, crispy types of fibers mechanically irritate new villi. Second, enzymes and other chemicals present in many raw vegetables (they can be blended to a paste or puree, but still remain destructive) can produce a negative chemical effect, causing increased inflammation (as in cases of raw garlic and onions considered before).

This idea of having special foods for the damaged gut can be rephrased: "The dead gut requires dead food". It takes only several hours for villi to re-grow (even after their complete destruction in the duodenum). The problem is that many people with serious GI problems continue to consume wrong foods (or do not have enough chewing) with each meal or every day. As a result, their villi are not able to become strong, resilient and mature.

With a right approach (when no mistakes are made), maturation of villi can be achieved within 2-3 days. Then the person can make a gradual transition to slightly rougher foods.

Let us consider examples of foods that can be used when a person has an inflamed small intestine.

10.1 Squashes

The best friends for the inflamed villi are organic **squashes**, such as **kabocha, butternut** (also called **buttercup**), **pumpkins, golden squash** and others. Cooked or baked squashes almost melt in the mouth and are easily transformed into a paste with tiny soft particles, which somehow manage to strengthen the inflamed villi.

Beware of tough fibers (which look like threads) that can be present near the skin or near the seeds of these squashes. These fibers should not be eaten. If you chew squashes well, the strings of these fibers should remain in your mouth.

Similar long fibers, but larger in their diameter, can be found in *spaghetti squash*. Even after very long cooking, this squash is not suitable for the anti-inflammatory diet.

Zucchini (also called courgettes) relate to squashes, and they have large seeds. However, if you cook zucchini for about 30-35 minutes, they become soft and can be easily chewed well (even with their green skin). Zucchini are almost as good as other squashes, but require good (but not long) chewing.

Note that long storage can change fibers in zucchini and make them or their skin unsuitable for this diet.

10.2 Root vegetables

Among organic root vegetables, some can be made very soft by long cooking. For example, after 30 minutes of cooking, **parsnips and rutabaga** become soft enough and suitable for the inflamed villi, if they are chewed well, and if you do not swallow tough fibers that can be present in these foods.

Potatoes, sweet potatoes, and yams are examples of starchy root vegetables that are possible to use for the anti-inflammatory diet. Make sure that you chew them well and remove all tough thin fibers. These fibers are often present in sweet potatoes and yams.

Very long cooking (over 40 minutes) makes ***carrots*** soft, but not soft enough for the anti-inflammatory diet. It is possible to make a paste from cooked carrots. However, since this paste includes starches, it requires good chewing. This is not easy to do when you already have a paste-like substance. As a result, carrots are not among the suitable foods.

You can only eat cooked fiber (pulp from a juicer) from carrots after you make a carrot juice. However, raw carrot juice has quite a large amount of fructose and cannot be used as a part of the anti-inflammatory diet. (Cooking carrots transforms their glucose into starches.) Therefore, the only option is to get a raw, nearly dry pulp of carrots after using a good juicer and cook this pulp for 1-2 minutes.

10.3 Nuts and seeds

Organic nut- and seed-butters are great for the anti-inflammatory diet. This relates to smooth butters made from organic **almonds, cashew nuts, sunflower seeds, sesame seeds**, and other nuts and seeds. Always read the labels and make sure that these butters do not have simple sugars (fructose, glucose, etc.) or cane sugar added.

Even crispy types of nut butters are usually appropriate since making these nut butters involves very high mechanical pressure that shear nuts and seeds mechanically, making them more susceptible to actions of digestive enzymes (provided that you chew crispy nut butter very well).

No matter how long you chew raw or roasted organic almonds, cashew nuts, or sunflower seeds, they will remain unsuitable for the anti-inflammatory diet. The same is true for pumpkin seeds, sesame seeds, linseed (flaxseed), and many other seeds. But when in forms of nut or seed butters, they are acceptable.

Organic smooth and crunchy peanut butters can be used as well, if you have no allergies to peanuts.

10.4 Grains and other starches

Starchy foods require very good chewing. In fact, among all types of foods, starches are the least suitable for the anti-inflammatory diet due to their nearly unavoidable negative effect on the inflamed villi. However, with very good chewing and presence of right other foods, this negative effect of starches can be minimized. And when we apply several additional positive factors, while avoiding all triggers, the GI recovery is easy to achieve, success even with some grains and other starches in the diet. If you do not have time and/or patience for chewing starches, you can explore diets that exclude grains and other foods with a high starch content.

The main digestion of starches should take place in the mouth due to the action of ptyalin. Let us consider specifics related to different types of starchy foods.

No matter how long you cook organic **brown rice or white rice**, it still remains chunky, and the small bits of skin of rice grains will damage the inflamed villi. There are different options.

- You may try to buy **rice cakes** (with no simple sugars added). However, many types of rice cakes have too many rough or tough pieces that are still present even after long chewing. These pieces cannot be transformed into a homogeneous paste in your mouth even after 150-200 chews. In some cases, a different batch of the same brand or a different brand of rice cakes can be suitable. Therefore, you may try to test and explore these options.

- You can make **bread from organic brown rice** flour. This flour can be found in large health food shops. To make bread, you will also need no-aluminum baking powder. However, if you make such bread in an oven, it may not be easy to chew and successfully digest its crust. The better option is to make the dough in a small stainless pot and put this pot for about 40-45 minutes in a larger pot with boiling water. Make sure that the piece of dough is no more than 3 cm thick. If it is too thick, it requires longer cooking time to cook all the way through.

- You can make brown rice porridge from **brown rice flakes**. Brown rice flakes (crushed rice grains) are available in many European countries, but rare in North America. Cook them for 10-12 minutes and then chew this porridge very well. Do not use too much water. In fact, you need to use as little water as possible, just enough to make some water available for all rice flakes. Then you will have better chewing and digestion of rice flakes.

There are different "cleaner" ways to cook rice flakes apart from simple boiling with water since the porridge can easily burn at the bottom even after 2-3 minutes of cooking. In fact, you do not need any boiling for rice flakes. Just boil water in a stainless steel pot. Then add rice flakes and immediately wrap the whole pot in a blanket (or jacket) to keep it warm for 10-15 minutes.

Alternatively, if you have a microwave, you can boil water in a glass or ceramic jar. Add rice flakes, close the lid, and wrap the jar in a blanket.

Making porridge from grains is a good option in relation to starches since this method allows you to make them soft enough for digestion and dry enough for longer chewing. Using saliva, rather than water, makes them more digestible.

Nearly the same ideas (as above for brown rice) are true for **buckwheat**. If you cannot get buckwheat flakes (e.g., you are located in North America) to make a porridge, you can easily make buckwheat bread, better in a plastic container, as described above.

Corn also requires tricky techniques in order to be a part of the anti-inflammatory diet.

- You can soak organic unsweetened corn flakes in water for at least 15 minutes to make them soft (when dry, they are crunchy and, even after good chewing, they damage the inflamed villi). Put corn flakes in a jar or container that can be sealed. Add a minimum amount of water just to make all surfaces of corn flakes wet. Invert the jar every 1-2 minutes to distribute water more homogeneously. In about 15 min corn flakes become soft (and not crispy on your teeth - just try them). Eat them while chewing very well.

- You can buy organic polenta and chew it very well.

- You can make organic polenta or corn bread from fine corn flour. (Do not use medium or coarse corn flour.) Mix fine corn flour with baking powder in a glass jar. Add hot or warm water (but not too hot) to this jar. Put this jar in a pot with boiling water. (The glass jar may stay on the bottom of this pot, with most part of the jar covered in water.) Medium-size and coarse corn flours have a tendency to settle at the bottom and their particles are too large (they will worsen inflammation).

You can cook corn without baking powder, but then you need to stir the mixture each 20-30 s while cooking in order to prevent settling. At a certain moment, the mixture becomes hot and nearly solid. Then you need to cook it for about 45-50 minutes. (Some varieties of organic corn can be pre-cooked and require less cooking. Read the label for these details.)

Remember that, as a part of the anti-inflammatory diet, we avoid *gluten products*. Therefore, all *wheat and rye products* are to be avoided. **Oats** have proteins that are similar to gluten and may cause a comparable damage for the inflamed villi. There is still no conclusive evidence in relation to effects of oats on the inflamed gut or people with sensitivity to gluten. Once you have achieved some success, you may check the effects of oats yourself. Maybe you can achieve no soiling while eating organic oat porridge.

10.5 Meats, fish and eggs

These foods do not require good chewing. However, it is better to eat them first or separately from starches following food combining ideas described below.

Note that conventional meat and eggs have reduced quality in North America and Australia due to use of hormones and antibiotics.

European animal products are generally of higher quality. However, for faster GI recovery, whatever your location, it is better to use only organic animal products.

Keep in mind that due to pollution of oceans and seas, nearly all **fish** has some mercury and other toxic chemicals. It is better to be vegetarian to avoid this problem and other problems associated with animal proteins.

Wild fish is much better, in comparison with farmed types of fish, such as salmon, due to higher content of EFAs (essential fatty acids) and better nutritional value. Smaller fish, like herring and sardine are virtually never farmed. Also, keep in mind that large, longest-living, carnivorous fish in the ocean, such as salmon, tuna, and swordfish, accumulate more toxins than smaller and younger types of fish.

Avoid conventional **eggs**, especially if you live in North America. Organic free-range eggs have much better nutritional value and less toxic and dangerous chemicals.

With higher CPs, people naturally eat less animal proteins. With over 40 s morning CP, many breathing students have no desire to eat meat and fish. This occurs due to improved metabolism of proteins.

10.6 Dairy and soy products

We have previously discussed the effects of dairy and soy products on the damaged GI system. Amongst all dairy products, butter has the smallest casein and lactose content. However, even very small amounts of protein in butter can cause GI problems, especially if you eat large amounts of butter. In any case, if you decide to eat butter, it is better to eat organic butter. This is particularly important for people living in North America.

We have also discussed above that, among soy products, only unsweetened organic soy yogurt might be suitable for the anti-inflammatory diet. If you decide to eat it, you need to closely monitor the effects of soy yogurt on urination and other GI signs.

Most types of tofu are usually impossible to transform into a homogeneous paste in the mouth. Even though tofu is a fermented food, it still can have a negative effect on the inflamed villi (experience of my students validates this). One may blend tofu into a paste and try it. Experience of my students suggests that it is still has a negative effect.

10.7 Beans and lentils

Since lentils and beans have a high content of starches, they require good chewing. The main problem with beans and lentils is their tough skin. The interior part gets soft after cooking, but the skin remains unsuitable for the anti-inflammatory diet. There are, however, some solutions.

Red lentils are sold without skin. They can be used for the anti-inflammatory diet. In some European countries, you can also buy **green lentils without skin**. This is how they are sold there. Cook them for about 15 minutes, or until they become very soft. However, if you use too much water, red and skinless green lentils become mushy, and there is a strong tendency to chew them less. To avoid this problem, do not try to cook them for a shorter time. If they remain a little bit hard (so that you cannot squeeze them with your tongue only), they will worsen inflammation in the small intestine. The ideal solution is to have a minimum amount of water so that they become very soft, but dry at the same time. Then you will chew them longer naturally. How to cook red or skinless green lentils with the least amount of water?

From the technical viewpoint, the "jar-cooking" method that was described above for making polenta is the optimum solution to make red or skinless green lentils very soft and dry at the same time. Fill 2/3 of the glass jar with red or skinless green lentils, add pure water (almost up to the top of the jar), and close the lid tight. Then put this closed jar inside a pan filled with warm or hot, but not boiling water. (Boiling water can break a cold glass jar due to a large temperature gradient.) The main part of the jar should be covered from outside with water. The jar may stay on the bottom of the pan or float there.

Once the water in the pan starts boiling, heat starts to slowly penetrate inside the jar. For this method, you may need to cook them longer (about 20-25 minutes of boiling instead of 15).

Green and brown lentils with skin are not suitable for the anti-inflammatory diet, even if you cook them for a very long time. The same is true for many types of **beans**. Even after cooking for 2 hours or longer cooking (some types of beans require even longer cooking - search the internet for instructions), their skin is still unsuitable for the inflamed villi.

However, you can buy **cooked lentils and beans**. The skin of lentils and beans from cans and jars is usually soft, but not because of longer cooking. It becomes soft probably due to long soaking in water after cooking (or they were cooked at high pressure). However, you must buy those cooked lentils and beans that are sold in jars, not in metal cans. Any type of food in metal cans should be avoided due to penetration of metals from the can into the food. Also read the label and make sure that they do not have simple sugars or strong spices added.

10.8 Berries

Berries are probably the most beneficial single type of foods for achieving a higher CP and better health due to their high antioxidant content and other benefits. However, nearly all berries have too much sugar for the anti-inflammatory diet. Their typical sugar content is about 6-9% even though they may not taste sweet. This is true for blackberries, raspberries, black and red currants, strawberries, blueberries, and so forth. As a result, most berries promote Candida in those people who already have inflamed villi. Another problem for people with GI problems in the small intestine is that many berries have very tough indigestible seeds. **Blackberries and raspberries** are examples.

Blueberries, currants, and strawberries have softer seeds, but their seeds are still too rough for the inflamed intestine.

However, powdered **Acai berries** have small particle size. This powder is soft enough and does not contain much sugar (less than 2% in raw berries or several times less than most other berries). This powder can be found in large organic shops in North America or can be ordered online. Organic freeze-dried varieties of Acai powders would be a good choice.

10.9 Fruits

Due to the presence of simple sugars, most fruits are not suitable for the anti-inflammatory diet. However, avocado has a very small content of simple sugars, and ripe avocados are fine for the anti-inflammatory diet.

Later, when the states of the villi and gut are improved, soft raw fruits can be used provided that the person has exercise with perspiration. This relates to ripe organic papaya, mango, peaches, kiwi, honeydew, some varieties of apples, pears, and other fruits.

10.10 NutriBullet for the soft anti-inflammatory diet

NutriBullet is a powerful (600 watts) blender produced by the same company that manufactures the famous Magic Bullet. The advantage of this blender is that it has 6 blades and more powerful motor in comparison with other blenders.

Ordinary blenders are generally unable to make vegetables, nuts and other foods suitable for the anti-inflammatory diet. However, according to experience of my students, NutriBullet is more effective and is able to chop and cut many raw vegetables into a paste that is acceptable for people with Crohn's disease, ulcerative colitis, IBS, and other conditions. This can be a great breakthrough in dealing with IBD since nearly all raw foods are not acceptable for the soft anti-inflammatory diet. However, one should keep in mind that, immediately after flare-ups, many raw vegetables can still be irritating due to their enzymes causing a laxative effect with increased inflammation. When

If this finding can be expanded on all people with IBD and IBS (that is very possible), then NutriBullet can become an excellent tool for their GI recovery. So far, it has been found that, with the use of NutriBullet, people with inflamed small intestine and ulcers can safely eat blended raw foods such as greens, broccoli, cauliflower, parsnips, sweet potatoes, zucchini, and many others. Even sauerkraut can be transformed into a paste suitable for people with IBD.

Limited experience suggests that the paste of raw vegetables, after partial recovery, has even a stronger healing effect on the damaged GI tract than squashes and other soft (cooked) foods.

11. Positive factors

After reviewing numerous adverse factors and triggers, you may get an impression that there are so many enemies that your chances of GI recovery are miniscule. In this Chapter, we are going to discuss numerous positive factors that can assist your GI restoration.

11.1 Breathing exercises

This book does not discuss the details of breathing exercises. However, it is important to know the general guidelines for breathing exercises for people with GI problems and inflammation of the small intestine.

We already discussed possible negative effects of some breathing exercises, and how breathing exercises can cause more inflammation and even mechanical damage due to presence of biofilms. These adverse effects of breathing exercises, when the exercises are done on an empty stomach, take place at about 20-25 s for the initial CP.

Since there are some individual differences, it is difficult to predict exactly and for all people if a certain person is able to safely perform breathing exercises. However, there are certain guidelines for those people who have inflamed villi and biofilms.

If you have less than 20 s for the current CP, you can push the CP up to about 25 s (or slightly less) by doing light breathing exercises. Having over 20 s CP is a crucial positive factor in GI recovery.

If you have about 25 s or higher CP, you should avoid breathing exercises, but do physical exercise with heavy or good perspiration in order to remove the biofilms and prepare the gut for more intensive breathwork.

Further details are provided in the next Chapter that discusses steps for GI recovery.

11.2 Earthing (electrical grounding of the human body)

Earthing has a known direct positive effect on any inflammation.
Chronic inflammation, according to new research, is a process that is
essentially controlled by an electric potential (abundance or
deficiency of free electrons) of the organism. This effect was
mentioned in the Section devoted to allergy tests.

Humans used to be electrically grounded to the Earth almost
constantly (due to barefoot life and absence of artificial fabrics and
shoes) just several generations ago, and this provided the human
body with a slightly negative electrical charge that corresponds to
Earth's negative potential. However, nearly all modern medical
research is performed on insulated humans and animals with a
positive electrical charge or electron deficiency. What are the
effects? Let us consider the key problem associated with chronic
inflammation.

In our current or popular understanding, inflammation is a response
of the immune system to injury. As a part of this response, the
immune system sends white blood cells to the site of injury. These
white cells include neutrophils that produce an oxidative burst in the
injured area. The neutrophils release reactive oxygen- and reactive
nitrogen species (also known as free radicals) in order to efficiently
destroy pathogens (bacteria) that usually penetrate across the skin
into the human body. This is a useful reaction that prevents
infections. These free radicals also break apart damaged cells so as
to rebuild healthy tissue and ensure healing. This process of
destruction is based on the chemical aggressiveness of free radicals
and their ability to "steal" electrons from other molecules.

Now we come to the main problem that causes chronic
inflammation. So far, these free radicals were doing a good job.
However, together with destruction of damaged cells and pathogens,
free radicals also leak into surrounding areas and destroy healthy
cells causing the classic quintet of hallmarks of inflammation:
PRISH or Pain, Redness, Immobility (loss of function), Swelling and
Heat. These classic features of inflammation are present in almost all

71

books on medicine and physiology. However, this (abnormal) scenario takes place in modern humans (and during animal studies) only in conditions of electrical insulation from the Earth and due to electron deficiency.

Grounding the human body to the Earth results in deactivation of free radicals in healthy tissues since the Earth can provide an abundant supply of electrons to neutralize free radicals, prevent damage of healthy cells, and "quench" chronic inflammation. As a result, grounding, within 10-30 minutes, reduces chronic inflammation and pain.

Therefore, the first and easiest step, in order to reduce chronic inflammation (that is one of the key factors in people with Crohn's disease, ulcerative colitis, and many other conditions), is to provide free electrons for the body using Earthing (the name of the technique). This will ensure those natural conditions that existed for millennia during human evolution.

In conditions of electrical insulation, lasting inflammatory problems often exhaust the adrenal gland that produces cortisol. Since cortisol is fundamental in reduction of inflammation and immune function, chronic cortisol deficiency makes CP growth impossible. Breathing students with too low cortisol get stuck, usually at about 12-15 s CP, and cannot progress further with breathing and physical exercises, however hard they try.

The solution suggested by Dr. K. P. Buteyko and his colleagues is to provide cortisol supplementation. However, in many cases, a faster and more natural health restoration can be achieved with Earthing.

How to ground yourself (Earthing)

You can ground yourself during daytime and/or sleep using simple DIY methods and techniques that can be found on this page: http://www.normalbreathing.com/e/how-to-ground-yourself.php. You can also buy commercial products (for example, an Earthing Mat or grounding sheets for sleep) online.

11.3 The "perspiration-breathwork" method

As we discussed before, if you have about 22-25 s CP and inflammation in the small intestine (with biofilms on its surface), nearly any breathing exercises lead to flare-ups. Even a mild CO2 increase produces damage to inflamed villi. At the same time, higher CPs is the most natural way to eliminate pathogens from the gut. What can be done to solve this challenge?

In such conditions, the solution is in the "perspiration-breathwork" method. If you do physical exercise with good perspiration, the state of your small intestine will be dramatically improved. There is no need to do very long physical-exercise sessions (such as 3 hours or more). If such sessions are intensive and long, they can be quite exhausting.

Find the balance and apply right-exercise sessions in order to clean your small intestine. If you sweat profusely and do about 1.5-2 hours of physical exercise, then later you can do intensive breathing exercises without any negative effects and quickly achieve much higher CPs.

Correct physical exercise provides the following benefits for GI health:

- mechanical vibrations of the human body cleanse the lymphatic system and intensify metabolism

- mechanical vibrations of the GI organs assist recovery of villi and other tissues due to increased blood flow

- perspiration removes toxins and, therefore, produces a relief for Peyer's patches in the gut helping removal of the biofilms.

These factors provide the foundation for the perspiration-breathwork method. Later, or in the long run, there is no need to have extensive concentrated exercise sessions. Daily physical exercise can be divided into smaller sessions. However, even after you made this step forward (and now can do nearly any breathing exercises), exercise starts to play a key role in your further CP growth.

The effects of physical exercise depend on its intensity and duration. Ideally, it is better to do more intensive exercise but with nose breathing only.

11.4 Duration of physical exercise

This Table reflects effects of duration of exercise on your next morning CP.

Duration of physical exercise per day	Maximum body O2 expected
0 min	15 s
30 min	20 s
60 min	25 s
1 hour of devoted PE + 1 h others	30 s
1.5 hour of devoted PE + 1 h others	35 s
2 hours of devoted PE + 1 h others	Up to 2-3 min

Table note. "1.5 hour of devoted PE + 1 hour others" means that the person spends, for example, 1.5 hour on devoted PE (physical exercise), e.g., 2 daily jogging sessions of 45 min each, and also gets 1 hour of walking here and there, in total, throughout the day.

Other explanations for the Table

Many sick people, especially city dwellers, often have about 20 min of physical exercise per day. (These 20 minutes include walking within the house, to the car, while shopping, etc.). Their body and brain oxygenation in the morning is, at best, according to this Table, about 18 seconds. This happens due to habitual chest breathing, possible mouth breathing and chronic overbreathing (breathing more than the medical norm at rest). This low body-O2 content makes GI recovery nearly impossible. Medical drugs may kill some pathogens, but are unlikely to provide a certain long-term relief.

If a person with over 20 second CP (Control Pause or body-oxygen test results) devotes 1 hour to rigorous physical activity with nose breathing only, he or she can get stabilized, over a period of some days, at the level of about 25 seconds of body O2. Usually people with nearly 20 s MCP (morning CP) have about 30 min of light exercise throughout the day (e.g., walking here and there). This is still insufficient for natural GI recovery.

Having more than 2 hours of daily physical activity is generally sufficient to get or maintain any body-oxygen level. This number should also be a target for people with GI problems.

Elderly people often require less physical exercise than suggested by this Table. For example, a 60+ or 70+ years old person may require only 1 hour of devoted exercise and 1 hour of walking to get any body oxygenation, provided that there are few, if any, negative effects due to other lifestyle risk factors.

Teenagers and young people in their 20s and 30s sometimes may require more physical activity to achieve main benefits of physical exercise and the corresponding body-O2 numbers shown in the Table.

Note that it is assumed here that, for getting higher CPs, other factors, including breath-work, sleep hygiene, diet, nutritional deficiencies, thermoregulation, daily work, and posture, do not produce negative effects on morning oxygenation. The same relates to various lifestyle factors related to digestion. In other words, it is necessary to avoid flare-ups to get morning CPs of 25 s and larger.

The situation for people with more serious chronic digestive diseases (as well as other accompanying conditions) is often worse. This means that people with physiological conditions or pathological tissue changes (inflammation, tumors, diverticula, strictures, deposits, lymphomas, granulomas, and so on) generally cannot get even 25 s for morning oxygenation without additional physical exercise.

11.5 Mechanical vibrations of the body during physical exercise

The anti-inflammatory diet requires soft foods in order to repair inflamed villi. Inflamed villi can tolerate only minimum amount of mechanical and chemical stress. As a result of low or minimum stimulation, one of the expected negative effects of such a soft diet is clogging of the villi with mucus and ingested food paste.

In order to remove excessive mucus, it is necessary to provide suitable mechanical stimulation. Such stimulation naturally takes place during many forms of physical exercise. For example, ordinary walking and jogging provide such mechanical stimulation.

There are different levels of intensities of body vibrations (shaking) due to exercise. Some forms of exercise provide very intensive (nearly maximum possible stimulation of body organs), while other activities are more gentle. Here are examples of physical exercise that are listed in an order, from gentle to more vigorous:

- Using an exercise bike; riding a bike on a smooth road (without large bumps, cracks, and other irregularities)

- Riding a bike on a bumpy road; slow walking with an empty stomach on an even (i.e., horizontal) surface

- Power walking on an even surface with an empty stomach

- Slow and gentle running on an even surface; power walking up and down the hill (all with an empty stomach)

- Nearly normal running on a soft surface (such as grass, small gravel or sand); fast walking downstairs and upstairs (all with an empty stomach)

- Nearly normal running on a hard surface (such as concrete, asphalt or rock); gentle running downstairs and upstairs

- Jumping rope (or skip rope) exercises; running 100 m dash; playing basketball and other games (all with an empty stomach); walking on an even surface with food or water in the stomach.

Note that the type of your shoes is an important additional factor if you do running on a hard surface. Some sport shoes greatly reduce the force of the mechanical impact that is experienced with each step, while other types of shoes (such as keds and sandals) do not make large difference on the force of the impact.

Usually, people with undamaged GI organs (or ordinary people) can tolerate the most intensive types of mechanical vibrations of the body. Depending on the type of the GI damage and its current state, a person with GI problems may not be able to do many or nearly all activities listed above. This particularly relates to more severe cases due to duodenal ulcers and IBD.

(Note that we do not discuss here the most severe cases of damage to digestive organs that leads to punctures, rupture, internal bleeding, and other serious traumas). Such traumas can take place due to car accidents, falling from high heights, and so forth. These types of damage often lead to inability of the GI system to digest any food. Such cases are handled in hospitals using total parietal nutrition, with nutrients delivered directly into a vein. Anything that is less damaging could be solved using ideas presented in this book.)

11.6 Positive effects of massaging devices and vehicle riding

However, in some cases, even very light forms of physical exercise with shaking are poorly tolerated. This relates to cases when the digestive organs are damaged almost as intensively as in cases that require total parietal nutrition. What are the solutions?

You probably have seen or maybe experienced **massaging chairs**. In addition, there are **massaging seating devices** (car seats), **massaging heat cushions**, and various **electrical massagers**. They can cost from about 20 up to 150 USD (for Shiatsu Massage Cushions).

As soon as these massaging devices have motors that create high frequency vibrations, they are beneficial for the body. Dr. K. P. Buteyko pointed out positive effects of vibrations on the human body many decades ago.

Such devices can be used for many hours every day after and/or during meals and even during sleep. These devices can speed up recovery several times and in severe cases can be life-saving. They are particularly beneficial for those people who cannot walk due to damage to GI and/or other body organs. However, even people with mild damage to the GI organs, as well as those people who cannot jog can benefit from their application.

The most intensive types of mechanical vibrations can be achieved using **whole body vibration machine**s that have become popular during last 1-2 decades. These machines provide intensive stimulation and can be used by some, but not all people with GI problems.

A similar (and sometimes even better) effect is present during **vehicle riding**. If a person with GI problems spends 2-3 hours in a moving vehicle (such as a car, bus, or train) or plane, this can lead to a faster GI recovery. This factor often speeds up GI restoration several times. It is not even necessary to experience or feel these mechanical vibrations. Many types of vibrations can be beyond human perception, but mechanical waves are absorbed by body tissues and villi helping their recovery.

There were cases of people who could not walk fast due to severe GI problems. However, after long trips in cars, trains or buses (up to 2-3 days), they achieved no soiling and could do running on a hard surface without any problems.

To be accurate, one does not even need a vehicle to move. This effect is present mainly due to high-frequency vibrations created by the car engine and not due to bumps on the road. Therefore, you can simply sit in a vehicle that has its engine working, and this will greatly assist repair of villi, removal of the biofilms, lymphatic drainage and other positive effects.

11.7 Food combining

The human digestive system is not well designed to digest mixtures of certain foods, especially at lower CPs. This is particularly true for mixtures that contain concentrated starches (such as grains, corn, buckwheat, and so on) and concentrated proteins (such as meat and fish). For example, if a person eats meat and rice (while mixing these foods together in the mouth), the stomach will experience a biochemical stress. The same is true for potatoes and fish eaten together and many other mixtures.

Why does it take a much longer time for the stomach to digest these specific mixtures? The effect takes place due to nearly opposite requirements for digestion of concentrated starches and proteins. Proteins require increased acidity (lower pH in the stomach) and more stomach enzymes in order for the GI system to successfully split proteins on peptides and polypeptides. Starches are not digested in the stomach to any significant degree. They are digested in the mouth due to actions of ptyalin and in the duodenum in a more alkaline environment.

As a result, the appearance of such complex mixtures (starches and animal proteins together) in the stomach makes the stomach "confused" resulting in much longer digestion. For many people with less than 20 s CP, such meals can remain in the stomach for more than 3 or 4 hours.

Among animal proteins, this effect is strong for meat and fish, but it is also present, in a smaller degree, for other animal products, such as cheeses and eggs.

What are the solutions? There are 2 main options.

One option is to eat these poorly compatible foods separately from each other (during different meals). We can call this method a **radical food combining**. You can eat animal proteins separately with vegetables (and fruits if they are suitable for you), but with no grain and no other concentrated starches such as bread, potatoes, corn and buckwheat. Starches can be eaten with vegetables during the following meal. Then animal proteins and starches are separated since they are eaten during different meals.

Another option is to eat foods in a certain order. We can call it a **partial food combining**. Here is an example. You can eat meat and fish first. Then you can eat vegetables, while chewing them well. Finally, you can eat starches at the end of the meal, while chewing them very well. What are the effects? If during this meal you do not drink too much water while walking around, the foods will be digested in the same order as you eat them. Animal proteins will be digested first. For the first portion of the meal, the stomach will be able to produce more hydrochloric acid for digesting animal proteins. Later portions of the same meal will get less acidic environment. This is not a problem, since later foods do not require an acidic environment and stomach enzymes.

As an overall effect for both types of food combining, you will spend much less time on digestion. As a result, you will have easier breathing and higher CP for a larger portion of the day.

11.8 Use of probiotics

There are certain types of beneficial (also called helpful) bacteria that should be naturally present in the large intestine in order to ensure good digestion and health. Some key functions of beneficial bacteria are:

- fermentation of carbohydrates and their absorption

- suppression of pathogenic microbial growth

- improved immunity

- syntheses of vitamins, such as biotin and folate

- help with absorption of ions such as magnesium, calcium and iron

- prevention of allergies and inflammation.

In healthy people, the small intestine should be nearly sterile or without any bacteria. This is generally true for new born, but nearly all modern adults have numerous types of bacteria and fungi, including pathogens, in the small intestine (and often in the stomach too).

When a person experiences soiling and other symptoms of poor GI health, the situation is worse. There are many pathogens that can dominate both the small and large intestines. Prolonged domination of pathogens can lead to complete or nearly complete disappearance of beneficial bacteria. Diarrhea or frequent bowel movements worsen the situation.

Most people living centuries ago did not use and, in many cases, did not have any foods with probiotics or beneficial bacteria in their daily diet. These people were likely to suffer from occasional digestive infections and severe diarrhea due to, for example, food poisoning. Therefore, on some occasions, they likely experienced nearly complete disappearance of helpful bacteria from the large colon. How could they restore their digestive flora? The appendix was the likely source of helpful bacteria. The location of appendix (at the very beginning of the large colon) is most suitable for this purpose.

However, many modern people chronically have very low body O2 levels (less than 20 seconds) and, as a result, very poor health. People with low CPs often do not have sufficient amounts of beneficial bacteria in the appendix (or nothing at all).

These are the main reasons why use of supplements with probiotics became popular during last decades. We can also understand why people with low CP benefit from frequent or daily use of probiotics.

Meanwhile, this situation is not normal. High CPs (over 30-35 s) and a reasonable diet naturally suppress pathogens and promotes growth of beneficial bacteria.

Experience suggests that, if you have less than 20 s MCP (morning CP), you may need to use probiotics nearly every day. If you have between 20 and 30 s for your MCP, you may need probiotics about every other day. With over 30 s MCP, only occasional use of probiotics is necessary (for example, once in 5-10 days) depending on soiling and other GI signs. With over 50 s CP 24/7, there is no need to use probiotics.

11.9 A super mixture with probiotics, prebiotics and psyllium husks

Repopulation of the damaged gut with good bacteria is very important but often not easy. We already discussed, for example, effects of low CPs. There is one serious problem with use of conventional probiotics and foods that contain beneficial bacteria (such as yogurt, kefir and others).

Generally, nutritionists and even most doctors recommend probiotics in capsules, powders or from yogurt. However, it is also known from clinical studies that up to 99% (in many cases over 99.9%) of good bacteria cannot safely pass through the stomach that is designed, with its low pH and enzymes, to kill all types of bacteria. Out of 10-12 common strains of good bacteria (commonly used in supplements and present in fermented foods) only Lactobacillus Faecalis can safely pass through the stomach. But one is not enough. The gut needs other varieties of good bacteria as well.

Therefore, good bacteria in yogurt, powders and capsules have very low survival rate and poor efficiency. What are the solutions?

Some companies started to produce **enteric coated tablets and capsules** that are able to survive low pH and actions of enzymes in the stomach and pass through the stomach unaffected. When such tablets or capsules arrive to the duodenum, pancreatic enzymes (with high pH or in alkaline conditions) dissolve these tablets or capsules, which safely release good bacteria for both colons. Such supplements are 2-3 times more expensive, but much more effective.

The main problem with enteric coated supplements for people with the inflamed small intestine is that these tablets and capsules are large and solid. They aggravate inflammation. Generally, for a person with IBD, taking 1 or 2 tablets or capsules is not as damaging as eating raw vegetables. However, it is better to avoid this stress. How?

This solution was suggested by some of my Buteyko breathing students. They informed me that they could achieve no soiling by using one special mixture and better food chewing. (These students had only 20 s at this stage.) Later I suggested to use the same mixture to many other students, and virtually all of them reported either very little soiling or no soiling at all. It was generally true even for students with low CPs (about 20 s or less). The positive effects took place within 2-3 days.

What is in the mixture? Imagine a mixture of 3 powders: probiotics, prebiotics, and psyllium powder (the main component).

Probiotics is a mixture of several varieties of good bacteria.

Prebiotics include those types of fiber that humans generally cannot digest (unless one has over 90 s CP), but these kinds of fiber are the main food for helpful bacteria. Inulin is the most common example, while fructooligosaccharides are other types of prebiotic substances that humans cannot digest. These types of fibers are commonly found in vegetables. Here are some common vegetables and their inulin content: onions have about 2-6 %, Jerusalem artichoke 14-19 %, garlic 9-16 %, artichoke 3-10 %, chicory 15-20 %, and so forth. Cooking has some negative or destructive effect on the content of prebiotics, but even "dead" (i.e., cooked) onions, garlic and other vegetables still fight pathogens by providing food for good bacteria in the gut. (This is another reason to eat vegetables, especially if you suffer from GI problems.)

Psyllium husks or **psyllium powder** is the 3rd component in the mixture. Their role is to attract a large amount of water.

How does this mixture work? When such mixture is dissolved in water, it forms a collagenous structure (like a jelly) mainly due to an ability of psyllium husks to draw in a large amount of water. As a result, good bacteria remain hidden inside this water matrix formed by psyllium husks.

What are the exact effects of such mixtures? When the stomach senses that it cannot digest the largest particles (such as particles of psyllium powder or husks surrounded by water), the stomach pushes the whole mixture through the pyloric valve into the duodenum (the first part of the small intestine). As a result, probiotics bacteria can survive their passage through the stomach by hiding themselves in the matrix formed by psyllium powder, while inulin immediately provides food for good bacteria creating conditions, in the duodenum and following parts of the GI tract, for probiotics to grow and multiply 10s or 100s fold.

Sometimes, such mixture can be bought in health food stores. You can also order them online. **BowelBiotics+** is one of the brand names that use the same 3 powders.

One of the options is to make this mixture yourself. You should be able to find psyllium husks, inulin (or other prebiotics - just ask for them), and probiotics (better in powder form or in capsules) in pharmacies (in some countries) and/or in health food stores. Inulin or other prebiotics would be the component that is hardest to find (among those 3 ingredients). But even if you get only psyllium powder and probiotics (in any form: capsules, tablets, or powders), then by eating vegetables for the same or next meal, you can achieve about the same general effect.

What are the ratios for this mixture? For a single dose, you will need about 1 tablespoon of psyllium powder (70-80% of the total dry weight for the whole mixture), about 1/4 to 1/2 of a teaspoon of inulin or other prebiotics (15-25% of the total dry weight), and 2-4 capsules of probiotics (3-5% of the total dry weight). Mix all powders before dissolving the mixture in water. Prepare and drink the mixture at the end of your meal to reduce the destructive effects of the stomach.

When ordinary people, even with the CP of 15 s, use this super mixture 2 times per day and chew their food very well, they notice no soiling in about 2-3 days. Note that this relates to people without serious GI problems. However, with good chewing and avoidance of all triggers, most people with digestive problems can also achieve the same effect in about 2-3 days.

Note that chewing is a crucial additional factor in order to achieve no soiling. Here is another example. Compare these low-CP no-soiling good-chewing people (discussed in the previous paragraph) with other people who may have over 30 s for the morning CP. MCP 30+ greatly assists the digestive flora in the gut. However, when such people do not chew food well, they may need to use the mixture again and again, maybe about 1-2 times per week or more depending on what they eat, and other factors.

11.10 Holding urine

As we discussed before, in adults, a healthy urinary bladder can hold about 1 liter or more of urine, while people with digestive problems frequently experience problems with frequent urination and reduced urinary volumes due to mechanical pressure created by structural abnormalities.

In many cases, especially when a person made a mistake and got a digestive flare-up, holding urine is nearly impossible. However, if a person makes the right choices, he or she can naturally hold urine for much longer time. That allows natural normalization of organ positioning. The enlarged urinary bladder can push a prolapse or inflamed folds of the small intestine into their right places. This improves blood supply to all normalized parts.

If the same person rushes to the toilet to pee at a slightest discomfort, this positive effect will not take place. This can prevent GI recovery. Furthermore, it is beneficial even to hold urine for as long as possible. It helps to speed up GI recovery.

Let us consider suggestions related to holding urine. If you make right choices related to your GI health (no flare-ups) and you try to hold urine longer, then you are likely to experience several more urges during the next 3-5 minutes. However, if you overcome these urges, the desire to urinate usually disappears for about 1 hour or more. Later, the urge can re-appear again and, in many cases, it is possible to repeat the process with the same effect.

Apart from these considerations, holding urine naturally favors easier breathing. In other words, when a person holds his or her urine, he or she naturally reduces his or her breathing and accumulates more CO_2 and O_2 in body cells.

This does not relate to bowel movements. One clinical study discovered that holding one's stool makes breathing faster and deeper. This makes sense since constipation can be quickly released with the Buteyko Emergency Procedure: breath holding and reduced breathing.

Therefore, the general guidelines are simple: we need to postpone urination, but not bowel movements. Although generally correct, the last rule, related to bowel movements, has exceptions that we are going to discuss in the next Chapter, which describes the transitory effects that take place during GI recovery.

11.11 Taking a warm shower with soap

When we take a shower, we eliminate large amounts of toxins from the surface of our skin. This effect is much stronger when we use warm water and soap. Skin is the largest organ of elimination which is exceptionally important for good digestive health. Let me prove this important idea with the following example.

If a person was burnt in a fire and barely lived, he or she will be in a critical care (or Emergency Department) of a hospital. People can generally survive when up to 50% of their skin is damaged. This means that only the remaining 50% of skin can still detoxify the blood and eliminate unwanted and poisonous substances. One may think that 50% of the body's skin is more than enough to do the job. When 1/2 of the liver or kidneys are destroyed (due to mercury, petroleum products or medical drugs), we may not even notice this. However, when 1/2 of the skin does not function properly, the effects can be disastrous.

These people (with about 1/2 of skin burned) often die. And the main threat to their lives is ... kidney failure. When a large area of the skin is damaged, the kidneys are overburdened with removal of metabolic waste products and toxins.

Note that, if kidney function is reduced almost to 0 (as during kidney failure), the human organism can still survive for days since the skin can replace kidneys to some extent.

Taking a warm shower with soap every day and after each exercise with perspiration is an important factor in GI recovery. This means that, if you do exercise with sweating, it is very useful to take a warm shower with soap right after the exercise session.

11.12 Taking a cold shower

Taking a cold shower is an additional tool that helps to increase the CP and blood flow to GI organs. In fact, a cold shower mechanically pushes blood from the surface of the human body (the veins) to inside (arteries and arterioles). There are many other benefits of taking a cold shower every day. For example, it leads to increased concentrations of brown fat cells.

If your blood glucose level remains normal after physical exercise, then a cold shower can be used after exercise (together with warm shower described above).

Note that you should not take cold shower if your current CP is less than 20 seconds. For more details, benefits and important safety rules related to cold shower, visit the web page - http://www.normalbreathing.com/l-cold-shower.php.

11.13 Barefoot walking and foot stimulation

Dr. K. P. Buteyko and his colleagues suggested that barefoot walking is an important part of their breathing retraining program. These doctors did not know about Earthing (grounding of the human body to the Earth). As a result, Buteyko breathing doctors suggested that the key benefit of barefoot walking is due to massage of numerous nerve endings located on both feet.

We described Earthing before, and mechanical stimulation of feet has an additional positive effect on GI recovery. Sometimes, due to insufficient stimulation of feet, people with GI problems develop skin peeling and itchiness on their feet. In many cases, the itchy or peeling skin areas, if we investigate reflexology maps, correspond to locations of their GI abnormalities.

If you decide to walk on gravel or do some other intensive foot stimulation, start with about 1-2 minutes per day and do it in the morning. If you walk or run on a soft grass, begin with about 10-12 minutes per day before noon and gradually increase the duration. (If feet stimulation is done before sleep, it can keep you awake for 1 hour or even longer.) Later, you can do feet stimulation before 6 pm.

You can also use foot massaging slippers, foot massage mats and machines.

11.14 Anti-Candida diet and plan

Candida Albicanis is a fungi and pathogen that causes yeast infection. Candida can become the main pathogen in the biofilm on the surface of the GI tract. Candida yeast feeds on simple sugars such as table sugar, brown sugar, and glucose and fructose from fruits. Heated or pasteurized honey does feed Candida, but raw or cold-pressed varieties of honey do not. Raw honey and Xylitol are among those rare simple (sweet) sugars that do not promote Candida.

The main problems with Candida are that right actions can make you feel much worse and that it is present in a degree. If you make right choices and eliminate all foods that feed Candida, then you can experience a die-off reaction (also known as the Herxheimer reaction) due to release of powerful metabolic by-products released into the body. Vice versa, when the person starts to eat fruits and/or table sugar, the die-off reaction stops; the person feels himself or herself much better, but Candida continues to multiply and colonize new areas in the digestive system.

How can someone discover or test strength of Candida in the digestive system? Some people are able to notice that they get too sleepy after eating, for example, a banana or grapes. This is a very strong sign. Other people may have craving for sweat foods.

Since Candida is present in the stool of healthy people, it is not easy to diagnose it clinically or using medical tests. Biopsy from the duodenum is one of the methods used by gastroenterologists.

My suggestion to my breathing students is to have no fruits and other foods with simple sugars (except raw honey) for 3 days and observe GI symptoms: urination, soiling, and so forth. Of course, this 3 anti-Candida test can be effective if there are no other triggers of GI problems, such as tap water, non-organic foods, and many others. You need to eliminate other possible triggers in order to get reliable results.

With less than 25 s for the morning CP, it is very possible and common that a person is going to benefit from this 3 day anti-Candida test and have less symptoms in 1-2 days.

The nest step is to develop a program that include following factors:
- physical exercise with heavy perspiration (or hot yoga or doing light exercise in a sauna) since this is the most powerful single gut

detoxification method
- all other activities that increase one's morning CP
- elimination of simple sugars (except raw organic or wild honey).from the diet
- using grapefruit seed extract available in health food shops due to its potent antifungal properties
- addition of coconut products in diet such as creamed coconut (bricks), coconut yogurt, organic coconut oil, and so on since these products contain large amounts of caprylic acid, a powerful anti-Candida agent.

With over 25-30 s for the morning CP and good daily perspiration, over 90% of students are able to gradually resume eating fruits without soiling and other negative effects. More details about the transitory diet and gradual reintroduction of fruits are provided below.

12. Steps for GI recovery

Due to a diversity of individual factors, there is no single diet that can well serve each person. The situation for people with GI problems is even more complex due to allergies, sensitivities and other parameters. However, there are several methods that can be used to get rid of biofilms and to slow down the hyperactive gut.

As a first step, a person with GI problems needs to monitor and identify all possible triggers and test their effects. After such triggers are found, it is necessary to eliminate them and introduce those positive parameters and lifestyle changes that are discussed in the previous Chapter. What are the next steps?

With avoidance of triggers, one needs to push the CP up with right breathing exercises, correct physical activity and other beneficial factors.

12.1 Approximate guidelines for breathing and physical exercises

If you have less than 20 s for the current CP, you need to increase your CP up to about 22-25 s by doing breathing exercises with light air hunger or while using the Frolov or DIY breathing devices.

If you already have about 22-25 s CPs, physical exercise will be a better choice since it allows you to partially restore the inflamed villi, to remove the biofilms and to prepare the gut for more intensive breathwork and higher CPs. Therefore, do some physical activity with good perspiration using the perspiration-breathwork method described in the previous Chapter. To increase perspiration, you can wear warmer clothing (even a jacket or vest) either for the last part or the whole exercise session.

If the physical exercise session is long enough (e.g., about 2 hours) and with good perspiration, after this exercise session, you can practice reduced breathing with a strong air hunger without any negative effects. This strategy (the perspiration-breathwork method) helps to achieve fast initial GI recovery and much higher CPs (up to 30-40 seconds). At this stage, you can also start using long breath holds, maximum pauses or absolute maximum pauses safely.

Another option (a slower method for "lazy" people) is to have less physical exercise, but with more intensive application of other positive factors, such as prolonged mechanical vibrations of the body (using massagers or riding vehicles) and using the super mixture with probiotics, prebiotics and psyllium husks. Then you may need about 2-3 days to achieve no soiling with other signs of good GI health.

It is possible to slow down the angry gut without physical exercise while applying numerous other positive techniques and factors described in the previous Chapter. (However, in this case, one needs to be careful with eating. Even slight overeating can cause elevated blood glucose. This will eliminate all your achievement and nullify your efforts in a few minutes.) For instance, if you discovered that mechanical vibrations have a positive effect on your gut, then you can spend a day, for example, riding buses. Buy a daily pass for local transport, take interesting books or videos with you, prepare right meals for the whole day, and go travelling.

What is going to happen next?

12.2 Disappearance of symptoms of poor GI health

With a proper program (good chewing, correct physical exercise, use of the super mixture, and so forth) and no mistakes leading to flare-ups, most symptoms (such as soiling, foul smell of feces, bloating, burping, frequent urination, cold feet, low or poor mood, and many others) disappear within 1-2 days. The morning CP can increase up to 5-10 seconds. Among previously mentioned symptoms of poor GI health, only thick (yellow or white) coating on the tongue remains present for longer time.

This is an ideal scenario that is present only in a small number of people. It is more common for a person to discover noticeable improvements in symptoms after making correct changes. However, he or she can learn that there are some other triggers that are not addressed yet. Therefore, many people get some improvements, but they still need to find out what else is missing (or present) in their lifestyle and diet.

Elimination of some triggers allows a more detailed investigation of the hidden remaining causes. When you already made many right choices, the effects of remaining hidden factors and triggers are more noticeable. Therefore, do not get discouraged if you did not achieve a large success in a few days. Study what is missing and address these factors.

Note that due to the synergetic effect, presence and dominance of pathogens in the gut (and presence of biofilms) greatly amplifies negative effects of mildly negative factors, such as conventional foods (or not organic foods), tap water, and many other mild factors. This means that, for a person without GI problems, it is possible to achieve good digestive health (with no soiling), while eating conventional foods and even drinking tap water. However, for a person with existing GI problems, the same factors produce a much stronger adverse effect and often prevent their GI recovery.

Therefore, it is beneficial to review all possible causes and think which of them relate to you.

12.3 Transition to rougher foods

Once you have no soiling and other symptoms of good GI health, breathing and physical exercises start to play more important roles in your further health and CP progress. In the past, GI exacerbations were keeping your CP down. Now, after you got noticeable GI improvements, you can join the majority of breathing students in pursuit of higher body O2.

As about diets, it can be a challenge to decide what to eat during these transitory times. The problem is that, even with various medical tests, we still do not have all details related to the remaining digestive problems and current abnormalities present in your GI tract. Changes in the digestive system (such as inflammation and biofilms) are very fast. A recovered person can create damage and biofilms in minutes. The same person can eliminate the existing biofilms in hours. Nearly all medical tests are too slow to reflect these dynamic changes. These are the reasons why you need to pay very good attention to a variety of your symptoms and signs.

When someone has ulcerations in the stomach or duodenum, it may take up to 3 weeks, in the case of right recovery conditions, to repair this abnormality and safely eat nearly any raw food (with good chewing).

Mechanical then chemical stimulation

As we analyzed before, apart from allergic triggers, people with digestive problems also have adverse reactions to too rough fibers and many chemical substances such as substances present in spices, acids, and essential oils.

During the transitory period, when new foods are introduced, it is important to reintroduce mechanical and then chemical stimulation. Somehow, during the recovery period, the digestive organs can still be not ready to process many chemical substances. But once the GI system adapts to rougher foods and fiber types, the same chemical substances do not trigger any negative reactions.

In more practical terms, you should start eating rougher foods (such as cooked carrots, Broccoli, and Brussels sprouts, raw spinach, and so forth) and later introduce, for example, raw onions and not buffered vitamin C. Do not eat foods that are stronger chemically first.

12.4 Intermediate diets

As we discussed before, there are different types of fibers with different effects on the digestive system. Some fibers are very soft (or can be made soft by cooking), other fibers are rougher. The considered soft anti-inflammatory diet is based on softest types of foods that allow a recovery of inflamed villi. Once the biofilms are removed and villi are more resilient, the digestive system will benefit from having rougher types of fibers and foods.

The semi-soft anti-inflammatory diet

Once the gut is able to accept rougher foods, it is beneficial, for overall health, to include them in the diet. The semi-soft anti-inflammatory diet includes, in addition to soft foods, the following organic foods:

- cooked green or brown lentils and beans

- cooked carrots, Broccoli, cauliflower, cabbage, Brussels sprouts, beetroots, onions

- cooked (or raw) mushrooms (but some of them can be too rough due to tough strings)

- cooked brown rice and buckwheat (without hulls)

- cooked quinoa

- walnuts and pine nuts

- raw spinach, tomatoes (without skin), green lettuce, Iceberg lettuce, raw zucchini (or courgettes)

- and other foods that are not crispy (when you chew them) and can be transformed into a paste.

The semi-rough anti-inflammatory diet

The next step is to add even rougher foods such as:

- raw carrots, Broccoli, cauliflower, cabbage, Brussels sprouts, beetroots, onions

- raw or roasted cashew, cooked peanuts, and roasted chestnuts

- strawberries.

The rough diet

Finally, there are foods that are most challenging for the gut even after long chewing. The rough diet includes:

- raw or roasted nuts (such as almonds and hazelnuts), pumpkin and sunflower seeds

- berries with their seeds (rasberries, blackberries, blueberries).

People with ulcers may need to postpone eating these foods for some weeks until healing is complete. Therefore, their better choice is to continue the semi-rough anti-inflammatory diet or the semi-soft anti-inflammatory diet.

Dairy and gluten products should not be used for at least some months.

12.5 Reintroduction of fruits

As we previously discussed, simple sugars from fruits worsen GI health. It is better to avoid them when one is dealing with soiling and other GI symptoms and problems related to biofilms and inflammation in the small intestine. Later, when soiling disappears, with higher morning CPs (about 30 seconds) and perspiration due to physical exercise, one can gradually add fruits. However, for the transitory period, fruit consumption should be limited.

During recovery and later, how much fruits can a person tolerate? For many people with around 30 s morning CP and heavy daily perspiration (or it is even better to have 2-3 exercise sessions with sweating per day), 1-2 medium fruits per day will not cause appearance of soiling. More fruits may not cause problems for 1 or 2 days, but can cause decreased urinary volume and appearance of soiling on the third day or later. The negative effect of fruits starts from a certain amount of daily simple sugars and is accumulative. The morning CP and daily perspiration are key factors that predetermine safe amounts of fruits.

If one manages to break through 40 s morning CP (this is very rare for people with GI problems, but possible), he or she can double fruit consumption even while still recovering from GI problems.

It is often impossible to tell exact amounts of fruits which is safe to use for any specific situation. Your individual situation may require some experimentation, tests and (unavoidable) mistakes. However, once the results are clear, GI recovery is much easier. As the safest options, you can avoid fruits during the recovery period.

12.6 Common mistakes during the transitory period

During this transitory period, you need to closely monitor your symptoms and see how the body reacts to reintroduction of rougher foods and new foods. The transition (from soft to a more normal diet) should not make the gut worse. The common mistakes during this transition are:

- too fast transition to rougher foods

- insufficient chewing that immediately causes inflammation and flare-up

- eating by time (not when hungry)

- eating too much fruits

- overeating (even eating vegetables that has nearly no calories still can cause serious problems, if your GI system is not ready to accept food)

- walking with food in the stomach

- exercising with food in the stomach

- doing wrong breathing exercises.

You should not get increased frequency of urination and reduced urinary volume, ear buzzing, and many other symptoms of worsened GI health. One of the greatest danger, during the recovery period, is the following effect.

12.7 The avalanche effect

Technically speaking, many people, even with IBD, are able to have a quick transition (within 2-3 days) to semi-rough raw diets without any negative immediate symptoms. A previously restricted person may start doing jogging, eating previously-forbidden foods, and do other things that were not possible or safe for a long time. However, when the gut is still in a state of partial repair, it is easy, for people with ulcers and IBD, to get a digestive flare-up and go back to the point zero due to the "**avalanche effect**".

Here is an example. Inspired by own advances and with much higher CPs, a breathing student may become less careful in, for example, chewing. An appearance of a small inflamed area will be greatly amplified by raw foods (even if they are chewed very well). The same jogging, instead of being a powerful recovery factor, again becomes destructive for the gut. As a result of small initial damage (during the transitory period) due to insufficient chewing, a person can quickly regress to his or her previous state of poor GI health with soiling and many other symptoms.

Therefore, once you notice first negative signs of worsened GI health (meaning that some damage is done), you need to immediately return to the soft anti-inflammatory diet and make other changes in order to prevent further GI damage.

13. Transitory and unusual effects during GI recovery

When a person makes correct choices and is on the right track to better GI health (often with higher CPs), it is very common to experience various unusual symptoms and transitory effects. Let us consider these temporary signs and effects of digestive improvements.

13.1 Temporary constipation

When a person implements the right digestive program, it is common to have no bowel movements for up to 2-3 days. However, it takes a much longer time for the digestive and enteric nervous system to adapt to the new control mechanisms in relation to bowel movements. This makes sense since all previous months (or years), the GI system was functioning in a state of low oxygenation and chronic emergency with trying to remove waste products from the polluted gut. Now the situation is different, and the gut becomes an integral part of the healthier organism.

Therefore, during the transitory period, one of the frequent complaints of breathing students is constipation. The symptom can be particularly strong for the first bowel movement. This complaint is more common among those people who did not use fiber supplements in their diet.

To ease this temporary challenge (later bowel movements becomes much easier due to adaptation of the GI system), you can apply the following techniques:

- the Buteyko reduced breathing exercise for faster constipation relief

- fiber supplements or psyllium husks in diet

- magnesium supplementation (if you want to know more about magnesium, see the Major Nutrients Guide and 3-day test for nutritional deficiencies - http://www.normalbreathing.com/l-11-major-nutrients-guide.php)

- 1-2 tablespoon of raw honey per day.

Note that at higher CPs (30+, and especially 40+ s), people can comfortably hold stool for many hours without negative effects on their health and CP. They just feel that they can have a bowel movement right now (if they wish), but there is no urgency since the body is in a good control. Therefore, they can easily postpone their bowel movements for many hours until their desire is stronger or there is a more suitable situation.

The scenario for people with low CPs is very different. In cases of severe GI problems, many people experience fecal incontinence indicating a lack of control over the GI organs. Many of them are aware that, if they do not get into the restroom in 3-5 minutes, the results can be disastrous. Their desire to defecate can appear suddenly, while their control is very weak (or nearly absent).

13.2 Getting sleepy after meals

When digestive health is improved, it is common for some people to experience sleepiness after meals (when the stomach just got empty) even when they eat only until the first signs of satiety and chew food well. In these conditions, the main cause of sleepiness after the meal is their low CP. In a sense, the body craves higher CP and more oxygen in cells since they habitually continue to hyperventilate after meals. Therefore, the solution to this challenge is simple. They need to do the Buteyko Emergency Procedure or a short session (about 3-5 minutes only) with breathing devices.

Note that it is also common for ordinary people to get sleepy after meals while they still have food in the stomach. While the effect (or symptom) is the same (sleepiness after meal), the cause of this problem is overeating that was likely caused by insufficient chewing and habitual compulsive eating.

13.3 A blocked pyloric valve (due to a peptic or duodenal ulcer)

When they start to recover, people with gastric or duodenal ulcers can experience a spasm of the pyloric valve (it is also called pyloric stenosis that is more common in infants, but also occurs in adults). The stomach digests and propels a part of a meal, but keeps the remaining part of the same meal inside, for some hours.

The effect may not cause any pain, but there is a feeling of heaviness in the stomach. Breathing remains heavy for these hours and the person cannot do breathing and physical exercises.

The possible explanation for this effect is the built-in mechanism that provides the stomach and duodenum with rest to recover. (This symptom is likely to appear only during recovery).

The solution to this challenge is to chew your food well and to be very sensitive to the slightest sensation of satiety (to stop eating). If you eat 1-2 extra mouthfuls, they can remain in the stomach for many hours and will cause this big problem.

13.4 Mild heartburn

Another unusual and temporary symptom is a light heartburn that can occur only for 1-2 days after meals. Later, this symptom disappears.

There is no need to do anything special. This reaction probably signifies a transition to a different regulation of work of GI organs.

Note that not all people necessarily get this or some other symptom during GI recovery. This is true for temporary heartburn as well. The appearance of a certain temporary abnormal symptom usually relates either to a new state of the GI system (the digestive system reset its work and control mechanisms in new conditions) or to the signs of the cleansing reaction when some digestive organ experiences detoxification.

13.5 Intestinal gas due to separation of colonic fecal impaction

Temporary intestinal gas (present for no more than 2 days) can be a sign of separation of colonic fecal impactions from the walls of the gut. This sign appears either due to raw or rougher diets or intensive vibrations of the body due to exercise. Let us first consider the mechanism of formation of colonic fecal impactions.

Colonic fecal impaction can appear in people who have sedentary lifestyle with a diet that is based on junk foods with nearly no fiber and no vegetables (or these vegetables are very soft as for the soft anti-inflammatory diet considered above).

When the soft anti-inflammatory diet is already unnecessary, but the person continues to eat only soft foods, then he or she can accumulate fecal impaction on surfaces of the intestines.

To rephrase the same observation, when the gut is partially restored and villi are stronger and more resilient, soft diets have a tendency to clog the villi and folds of the gut with residues and mucus often causing formation of fecal impactions on the walls of both colons. There are several solutions to this challenge.

When the person starts **eating raw or rougher foods**, these rougher foods wipe away this fecal impaction. Therefore, if it is safe to eat rougher foods, then you should do it. The considered semi-soft anti-inflammatory diet is effective for this purpose. Eating raw papaya or pineapple is another effective method to get rid of debris formed in the small intestine due to the soft anti-inflammatory diet. (These fruits contain papain and bromelain that helps to do the job.)

Psyllium husk powder (but not fine ones) produces about the same positive stimulating effect on food residues. As we discussed, psyllium husks can be a part of the soft anti-inflammatory diet.

Mechanical vibrations of the whole body (as during jogging or due to massaging devices or vehicle riding) also help to mechanically separate fecal impactions from the walls of the gut. The effects depends on intensity and duration of stimulation.

13.5 Foam in the mouth or frothy saliva

When the body starts to repair inflammation in the stomach, it is common to experience white foam in the mouth (or frothy saliva). This symptom can be strong during physical exercise or breathing sessions. Higher CO2 favors easier removal of this foam from the stomach.

If there is no further damage to the stomach, this symptom also quickly disappears.

Apart from higher CPs, eating when hungry and other steps that have been described above help to speed up disappearance of this symptom.

13.6 Vomiting old bile

If a person had serious problems with his or her liver, and the composition of bile in the gallbladder does not fit his or her improved health (with higher CP), then the old bile and possibly other toxic and unwanted chemicals can be removed through the stomach. This is manifested in vomiting of old bile.

13.7 Feeling cold all the time (chill)

As it was previously discussed, some people with digestive problems are not able to safely run due to ulcers and other abnormalities in their digestive organs. As a result, in order to restore their health, they often do focus on gentle types of exercise, such as cycling, using exercise bikes and safe types of weight lifting.

When these people partially recovered their GI health and can safely start running, they can experience chill, a sensation of coldness, which is often accompanied by shivering and pallor of the skin.

This chill is a sign that the body is ready and even requires running to normalize metabolism, digestive health, circulation and other vital functions after long time of physical "semi-hibernation". Therefore, if you get this sensation, start running (on a soft surface) and later gradually increase duration and intensity.

14. Questions and answers

Q: I always have bowel movements in the morning with greasy stool. Why is this?

A: It is most likely that there is some GI trigger that causes a flare-up between your last daily meal and early morning hours. You need to review all factors and see what can be wrong in your lifestyle or diet. It may relate to your last meal, tooth brushing, and numerous factors related to sleep.

Q: Can people with GI problems use alcohol?

A: If alcohol does not cause a GI exacerbation, then, according to Buteyko, it should be limited by the morning CP number in milliliters. For example, if you have 20 s MCP, you can safely have 20 ml of pure alcohol for this day. If you morning CP is 40 s, you can use 40 ml of pure alcohol per day.

Otherwise, if you exceed this amount, alcohol can have a negative accumulative effect and gradually destroy your liver.

Q: Would having 50% percent of daily calorie intake (total of about 2,200 calories) come from one of three meals be an OK idea? Since I have time first thing in the morning, I'm thinking that I can use it to chew, getting a whole hour and a half to eat breakfast.

A: Some people indeed, have more hunger and can eat a lot for their breakfast. It is their normal lifestyle. Most importantly, eat when hungry and stop in time. You can even have only 2 meals per day.

Q: Even mild walking creates lack of saliva. Saliva becomes frothier than anything. Is it wrong?

A: Lack of saliva may indicate more inflammation in the colons, while frothy saliva is a likely sign of stomach detoxification. You can also have both at the same time. In order to be certain, monitor your urinary output, soiling, flatulence. Would long walking create more burping, and offensive intestinal gas? If yes, then walking causes problems. You can also try an exercise bike and see the difference.

Q: Do I ask the doctor for test to assess for ulcer or is there another way to diagnose? Is healing done through rest?

A: Endoscopy is the common way to diagnose ulcers. Rest will not help with biofilms and better GI flora. Healing is done through perfect chewing, right diet, right exercise, high CP, and other factors. Enough sleep and rest matters too, but this is not enough for success.

Q: Is there some guideline on how long to wait to do the Reduced Breathing after a given amount of food?

A: It is impossible to be 100% accurate. For an ordinary modern person, who has 3 large meals per day (breakfast, lunch and supper), an ordinary lunch or supper requires about 2.5-3 hours to pass through the stomach. However, if you have normal weight and do heavy labor all day (some people do this without breakfast and lunch), by supper time you will be super hungry and can digest an ordinary lunch or supper in about 20-30 minutes! Someone obese, on the other hand, with low CP, may need longer than the average time. As a result, there are many people who have food in the stomach all day long.

You need to develop a sense related to physical emptiness of your stomach. Pay attention to changes in your breathing, desire to exercise, and other physiological signs.

15. Conclusions and final remarks

As you may notice that this book suggests that science of digestion does not exist yet. Existing books on digestion do not have clear criteria of good (or normal) digestive health and do not provide clear and effective plans to deal with digestive problems.

This book is probably one of the first attempts (or maybe the first attempt) to explore this area. Feel free to leave your questions and comments on web pages devoted to digestive health:

http://www.normalbreathing.com/digestive-health.php

http://www.normalbreathing.com/how-to/how-to-improve-digestion.php

16. Recommended reading

You can also be interested in these books:

Free book (August 2013): "**Jump Start Your Gluten-Free Diet! Living with Celiac / Coeliac Disease & Gluten Intolerance**", by Kim Koeller, Stefano Guandalini MD and Carol Shilson: http://www.amazon.com/Gluten-Free-Coeliac-Intolerance-Allergies-ebook/dp/B00BF1NCM6/

For most people, it is nearly impossible to recover from Crohn's disease or ulcerative colitis, while having bread and other gluten products in diet.

Breaking the Vicious Cycle: Intestinal Health Through Diet [Paperback only] by Elaine Gloria Gottschall: http://www.amazon.com/Breaking-Vicious-Cycle-Intestinal-Through/dp/0969276818/

This is a great book for those who does not have enough time or does not have patience to chew starches very well. Then you can be better without any starches while applying the legendary SCD (special carbohydrate diet).

About the author: Dr. Artour Rakhimov

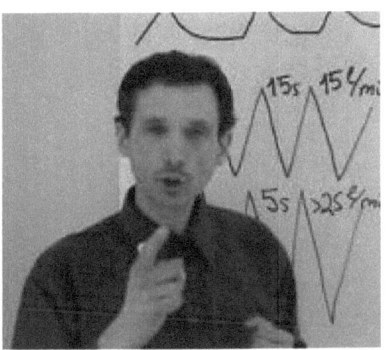

* High School Honor student (Grade "A" for all exams)
 * Moscow University Honor student (Grade "A" for all exams)
 * Moscow University PhD (Math/Physics), accepted in Canada and the UK
 * Winner of many regional competitions in mathematics, chess and sport orienteering (during teenage and University years)
 * Good classical piano-player: Chopin, Bach, Tchaikovsky, Beethoven, Strauss (up to now)
 * Former captain of the ski-O varsity team and member of the cross-country skiing varsity team of the Moscow State University, best student teams of the USSR
 * Former individual coach of world-elite athletes from Soviet (Russian) and Finnish national teams who took gold and silver medals during World Championships
 * Total distance covered by running, cross country skiing, and swimming: over 100,000 km or over 2.5 loops around the Earth
 * Joined Religious Society of Friends (Quakers) in 2001
 * Author of the publication which won Russian National 1998 Contest of scientific and methodological sport papers
 * Author of the books, as well as an author of the bestselling Amazon books:
 - *"Oxygenate Yourself: Breathe Less" (Buteyko Books; 94 pages; ISBN: 0954599683; 2008; Hardcover)*
 - *"Cystic Fibrosis Life Expectancy: 30, 50, 70, ..." 2012 - Amazon Kindle book*
 - *"Doctors Who Cure Cancer" 2012 - Amazon Kindle book*

- *"Yoga Benefits Are in Breathing Less" 2012 - Amazon Kindle book*
- *"Crohn's Disease and Colitis:* Hidden Triggers and Symptoms*" 2012 - Amazon Kindle book*
- *"How to Use Frolov Breathing Device (Instructions)" - 2012 - PDF and Amazon book (120 pages)*
- *"Amazing DIY Breathing Device" - 2010-2012 - PDF and Amazon book*
- *"What Science and Professor Buteyko Teach Us About Breathing" 2002*
- *"Breathing, Health and Quality of Life" 2004 (91 pages; Translated in Danish and Finnish)*
- *"Doctor Buteyko Lecture at the Moscow State University" 2009 (55 pages; Translation from Russian with Dr. A. Rakhimov's comments)*
- *"Normal Breathing: the Key to Vital Health" 2009 (The most comprehensive world's book on Buteyko breathing retraining method; over 190,000 words; 305 pages)*

* Author of the world's largest website devoted to breathing, breathing techniques, and breathing retraining (www.NormalBreathing.com)
* Author of numerous YouTube videos (http://www.youtube.com/user/artour2006)
* Buteyko breathing teacher (since 2002 up to now) and trainer
* Inventor of the Amazing DIY breathing device and numerous contributions to breathing retraining
* Whistleblower and investigator of mysterious murder-suicides, massacres and other crimes organized worldwide by GULAG KGB agents using the fast total mind control method
* Practitioner of the New Decision Therapy and Kantillation
* Level 2 Trainer of the New Decision Therapy
* Health writer and health educator

www.ingramcontent.com/pod-product-compliance
Lightning Source LLC
Chambersburg PA
CBHW050403290526
45786CB00003B/1112